Parents Whose Parents Were Divorced

R. Thomas Berner

The Haworth Press
New York • London • Norwood (Australia)

The Haworth Press, Inc., 10 Alice Street, Binghamton, NY 13904-1580

Library of Congress Cataloging-in-Publication Data

Berner, R. Thomas.
   Parents whose parents were divorced / R. Thomas Berner.
     p. cm.
   Includes bibliographical references and index.
   ISBN 1-56024-138-1 (alk. paper) — ISBN 1-56024-139-X (pbk.)
    1. Adult children of divorced parents — United States. 2. Parenting — United States — Psychological aspects. 3. Family life surveys — United States. I. Title.
HQ777.5.B48   1991
306.89 — dc20   91-6813
                                                             CIP

Parents Whose Parents Were Divorced

HAWORTH Marriage and the Family
Terry S. Trepper, PhD, Senior Editor

New, Recent, and Forthcoming Titles:

Christiantown, USA by Richard Stellway

Marriage and Family Therapy: A Sociocognitive Approach by Nathan Hurvitz and Roger A. Straus

Culture and Family: Problems and Therapy by Wen-Shing Tseng and Jing Hsu

Adolescents and Their Families: An Introduction to Assessment and Intervention by Mark Worden

Parents Whose Parents Were Divorced by R. Thomas Berner

The Effect of Children on Parents by Anne-Marie Ambert

Multigenerational Family Therapy by David S. Freeman

101 Family Therapy Interventions edited by Thorana Nelson and Terry S. Trepper

Therapy with Treatment Resistant Families: A Consultation-Crisis Intervention Model by William George McCown and Judith Johnson

For my mother,
who was also my father

ABOUT THE AUTHOR

R. Thomas Berner, MA, is Professor of Journalism and American Studies at Pennsylvania State University. He is a member of the Society of Professional Journalists and the Association for Education in Journalism and Mass Communications. He is the author of four books, *Language Skills for Journalists, Editing, Writing Literary Features* and *The Process of Editing*. A frequently invited guest speaker, he has spoken at over thirty journalism and writing seminars in the past sixteen years. Mr. Berner's interest in the issues of divorce stems from his own experience as a child of divorce who is now a parent. He received his MA in Journalism and his BA in English Literature both from Pennsylvania State University.

CONTENTS

Senior Editor's Comments

Few social problems affect so many of us as divorce. There is virtually no one in the United States whose life has not been touched by the sadness of divorce. We are only beginning to see the long-term social and psychological effects as the children of the first "divorce generation" are now adults and parents themselves.

There have been literally hundreds of books written about divorce: from the popular psychology/self-help books for the partners, children, and extended family, to books for clinicians on how to treat each of these sub-systems affected by divorce, to presentations of large empirical studies on the social, systemic, and psychological etiologies of divorce. However, few have tackled the difficult task of chronicling the phenomenology of divorce. That is, until now.

R. Thomas Berner, in his book *Parents Whose Parents Were Divorced*, captures the pain, sorrow, and eventual survival of those most traumatized by divorce: the children. In a thorough qualitative analysis, Professor Berner has captured the essence of the experience for almost 300 adults whose parents divorced when they were children. What is presented is extremely personal yet generalizable; simple in presentation yet profound in impact; poignant yet hopeful.

The book is wonderfully written. So many books that present the results of research studies are, frankly, quite boring to read. Not so in this case! Professor Berner, an experienced journalist and professor of journalism, knows how to present information in a clear, readable, and interesting way. This is especially fortunate; the results of the study are so potentially useful to so many different people, it would have been a shame to lose that by virtue of a pedantic presentation.

I believe *Parents Whose Parents Were Divorced* will be invaluable to teachers, researchers, students, and anyone who has lived through — and beyond — a divorce. I hope you enjoy it as much as I did.

Terry S. Trepper, PhD
Senior Editor
Haworth Marriage and the Family

Preface

What do we know about children of divorce who are now parents? What was life like for them? What do we know about those children who, because of their parents' divorce, were in the minority, who were treated differently by many of their friends and relatives?

What was their family life like during the divorce? Did they lose their friends after the divorce? How did they mature and what did they think of themselves?

In the face of economic and emotional deprivation, how did they face life with their custodial parent? Did they see their non-custodial parent regularly — or ever? Was there any attempt at reconciliation between the non-custodial parent and the children? Was it successful? When they became parents, what adjustments did they make because they had grown up in a divorced home? How do they parent? How did they get along with their spouse? Knowing what growing up in a divorced home was like, would they themselves divorce? What legacy does divorce leave?

We do not know much about children of divorce who are now parents. They have not been studied much. Attention has mostly been focused on young children just going through their parents' divorce or a few years after the divorce.

Parents Whose Parents Were Divorced focuses on children of divorce who are now parents by bringing together expert opinion on divorce and the testimony of children of divorce who are now parents: in other words, the testimony of adults who have lived through divorce as a child, grown up, married, and raised — or are raising — their own families. *Parents Whose Parents Were Divorced* answers the questions raised above.

And what do we learn?

We learn that, popular belief to the contrary, divorce does have a lifelong impact. We learn that divorce does not go away. It does not easily recede into the memories of children as they grow into adulthood. We also learn that children who grew up in a divorced home do not necessarily end up in reform school or prison. We learn that children of divorce can overcome the trauma. Today, some of them are secretaries, doctors, attorneys, and professors. Today, they are contributing to society. So, while we learn that divorce has an impact, we also learn that the impact is not always a negative or regressive one.

How does one probe the memories of adults who grew up in divorced homes and became parents? There are several ways. Working with limited funds, I chose a questionnaire.

My questionnaire contained open-ended questions meant to elicit personal responses rather than a range of responses that could be tabulated. I wanted to hear people talking about their experiences as children of divorce.

Since the questionnaire is included (see Appendix), readers who are children of divorce are invited to fill it out. (It takes about four hours.) Many respondents to my query reported feeling better after filling out the questionnaire. They said it removed a great weight or helped them develop a better awareness of themselves.

I pledged confidentiality to all respondents and agreed that I would use only general identification in whatever I write. All names in this book are pseudonyms for the respondents. Eventually, all returned questionnaires — whether used in this book or not — will be sealed and delivered to the Office of the Vice President for Research and Graduate Studies at The Pennsylvania State University to guarantee perpetual confidentiality.

In order to present this analysis of divorce, I combined many of the responses to my questionnaire with the findings of experts' research. The interpretations are my own. The voices belong to the children of divorce who are now parents.

Acknowledgments

This book could not have been written without funding. The sole supplier of it was the Office of the Associate Dean for Research and Graduate Studies in the College of the Liberal Arts of The Pennsylvania State University. I would like to thank the three deans who have occupied that office during the period of my fund searches: Thomas J. Knight (who has moved on), Thomas F. Magner (since retired), and Joseph W. Michels (who replaced him).

Another person in the research office who has my eternal gratitude is Irene Johnston (now Irene Johnston Petrick), the coordinator of grants and contracts. Irene worked patiently with me, a novice (and unsuccessful) national grant supplicant. When she realized that much of my preliminary work would come to naught without some funding, she persuaded Dean Michels to provide me with additional financing. Had she not done that, I would have had 459 letters from interested people but no money to send them a questionnaire.

The School of Journalism's administrative staff (at the time) of Christine L. Templeton, Patricia E. Kidder, Shelba J. Winfree, La-Dawn H. Dutrow, and Delores J. Vonada cheerfully coordinated, typed, and duplicated the questionnaire and the bulk of all correspondence. Further, Chris and Pat frequently expressed a personal interest in my work on "the divorce book" in a way that always gave me a lift. Eventually, a new secretary, Penny Snyder, joined us and, as a divorced mother of two young children, became an instant supporter of this book. She was followed by Stephanie Cunefare, who was equally supportive. Additional moral support came from Brian N. Winston, Dean of the School of Communications, which superseded the School of Journalism.

Another person who came up with the right stuff at the right time was my one-time journalism department head, R. Dean Mills. In addition to committing secretarial time to keep the project going, he also devised a teaching schedule that gave me four days a week to write. (Eventually, I needed a one-semester sabbatical to get the job done right.)

The research received some publicity from Kathleen V. Pavelko, who, at one time, hosted a public affairs show on Penn State's public television station, WPSX-TV. In the best scholarly tradition, she gave me a forum in which to discuss my ideas.

Former students deserve my thanks for clipping articles along the way or for discussing their own reactions to their parents' divorce. One student, Mike Rinker, did the initial bibliographic search in Penn State's library (before computers!), which saved me several weeks of work. Jack Pontius, an Associate Librarian and the library's liaison with the old School of Journalism, promptly filled all my requests for new books and put some orders on highest priority when time was of the essence.

My appreciation is extended also to the experts who corresponded with me. They asked good questions and they gave good direction. Some of them shared research ideas with me, even though we appeared to be working in the same area (but with different methods). Along with their affiliation at the time we corresponded, they are listed here in the order I wrote to them: Dr. Paul Bohannan, University of California, Santa Barbara; Dr. Herbert G. Zerof, Director, Family Therapy Center, Charlotte, North Carolina; Dr. Judith S. Wallerstein, Center for the Family in Transition, Novato, California; Professor Paul C. Glick, Arizona State University, Tempe; Professor Andrew Cherlin, Johns Hopkins University, Baltimore; Dr. Michael A. Smyer, The Pennsylvania State University; Professor C. John Sommerville, University of Florida, Gainesville; Ula Maiden, Mildred E. Strange Middle School, Yorktown Heights, New York (who, with John Brogan, teaches a course on divorce); Dr. Betty L. Moore, Student Assistance Center, The Pennsylvania State University; Dr. Michael S. Jellinek, Massachusetts General Hospital, Boston; Dr. Frank Furstenberg, The University of Pennsylvania, Philadelphia; Dr. Martin J. Schultz, The Pennsylvania State University; Dr. Louise Guerney, The Pennsylvania State University; Dr. Vladimir DeLissovoy, The Pennsylvania State University; Dr. Michael E. Lamb, University of Utah, Salt Lake City; Dr. Jerry M. Lewis, University of Texas, Dallas. Naming them here does not imply their endorsement of my work.

Prompt semantic help came from Professor Andrew Hacker of the Division of the Social Services, Queens College, New York, who is the author of *U/S*, an interesting and readable statistical look at the United States. Equally prompt forwarding of relevant statistics came from Dave Lewis of the U.S. Bureau of the Census.

I also want to thank the six people who formed the focus group in order to critique the questionnaire (one did it by mail). These six people immensely improved the content of the questionnaire: Gayle Flick, Centre Hall; Cyndi Barningham, Pleasant Gap; Frances Stevenson, Port Matilda; Wendy Williams, Port Matilda; Jeanette Janota, Lemont (all of Pennsylvania); and Nancy Johnson, Ruckersville, Virginia.

Designing the questionnaire was quite a challenge for me, an amateur. Professional help came from John S. Nichols and John V. Pavlik — colleagues who provided me with reading material on how to construct a questionnaire, especially one that the respondent would fill out on his own. Further, "Nick" always gave me his usual thoughtful feedback, almost from the day I conceived the idea for the book.

Two other people already cited also offered useful advice on the design and content of the questionnaire: Dr. Michael S. Jellinek of Massachusetts General Hospital and Dr. Vladimir DeLissovoy, Professor Emeritus of Child Development and Family Relations at The Pennsylvania State University.

I was very fortunate to be able to recruit a friend, Nydia Finch, to edit the book both for concept and context. (Her editing included trimming the length of my praise for her.)

I also want to thank my former wife, Karen, for her understanding in this project. As this book went to press, we coincidentally initiated divorce proceedings, having raised two daughters.

Finally, the daughters. Since I was raised without a father, I wanted more than anything to be a good father. I leave that judgment to Tracey and Amy. I do thank them for their love, which I hope is forever.

Methodology

To locate children of divorce who would be willing to fill out the questionnaire, I turned to daily newspapers. I knew that some newspapers in the United States routinely publish authors' queries free of charge. I sent my query to 316 daily and Sunday newspapers, from the *Advertiser-Journal* in Montgomery, Alabama, to the *Sunday Tribune-Eagle* in Cheyenne, Wyoming. Some editors went beyond the query and had reporters call me to write a story about my research. At least one such story, by Vickie Kilgore East of the *Tennessean* in Nashville, reached me.

Although not every newspaper published the query, I received letters of interest from 459 people in 39 states and the District of Columbia. Of those 459, 231 filled out the questionnaire. Some of them also provided me with the names and addresses of their siblings — 123 in all. Of that number, 36 filled out a questionnaire. I consider this outcome fairly good considering that I sent the questionnaire without warning.

Let me acknowledge some shortcomings. First, the people who responded to my questionnaire constitute a self-selected sample. Obviously, I reached people who, for the most part, had the confidence to put their thoughts on paper.

Based on my breakdown of the respondents, I did not reach many racial minorities or males. Long after collecting the questionnaires, I learned from an article that sons tend to create greater stability and thus diminish the possibility of a divorce.[1] Considered in that light, I am glad I received as many responses from males as I did. It also explains the number of female respondents and the indication that many of their siblings were female.

ENDNOTE

1. Morgan, S. Philip, Lyne, Diane N., and Condran, Gretchen A., "Sons, Daughters, and the Risk of Marital Disruption," *American Journal of Sociology*, Vol. 94, No. 1, July 1988.

Chapter One

Divorce

"A major marital status phenomenon in American society," according to the Census Bureau, "is not marriage but a continuing upward trend in divorce." Between 1970 and 1987, the divorce ratio almost tripled, from 47 divorced persons per 1,000 married persons to 130.[1] Since 1960, the ratio has quadrupled.[2] Two-parent households have been on the decline since 1949 when they represented 79 percent of all households. More recently, they represent 61 percent.[3]

Out of this rising divorce rate has come still another phenomenon – the one-parent household. In 1988, the number of children living with only one parent was 15.3 million.[4] Between 1970 and 1988, the proportion of children living with one parent doubled.[5] In roughly the same time, the Census Bureau reports that the total number of children under 18 dropped from 64 million in 1960 to 63 million in 1986; meanwhile, the number of children affected by separation and divorce continued to rise.[6]

Even more compelling is the prediction that this situation will get worse. One divorce scholar predicts that a high proportion of this country's more recently married couples will continue to divorce.[7] Another scholar says that the proportion of children who will live in a single-parent home is much larger than the number of adults who will be single parents.[8] "By 1990, 30 percent of all children will be in single-parent families," one family-oriented agency says. "Half of all children will have spent some time in a single-parent family before reaching 18."[9] In 1980, it was 20 percent.[10]

More married women than men will feel the impact of single parenthood. Women have a one in two chance of becoming a single parent; for men, it is less than one in 20.[11] One effect on women is

2

the loss of a male income.[12] "A high percentage of people in poverty are women raising children" says Bruce Chapman, the director of the Census Bureau. "Poverty seems to attach itself to people trying to raise children alone."[13]

What other deprivations can a child of divorce expect?

For one, good parental role models. It is not planned — this establishment of role models by married couples — it just happens. Parents do not realize that they are acting as models and children do not know they are learning to be fathers and mothers.[14] The use of attention and affection in this unconscious modeling process seems to be more important than food and physical caretaking.[15]

Out of this nurturing experience grows the individual's sense of family. "The manner in which we learn to behave and react in our family," says one researcher, "eventually molds our view of the world. In this sense, we re-create our family again and again in other environments."[16] One asks — rhetorically, for now — what kind of family does a child of divorce create?

And what does the two-parent family provide children? The answer comes from many directions. "In any marriage," one researcher says, "husband and wife achieve consensus and coordination."[17] There is a bit of bargaining in marriage[18] which the children see, unconsciously absorb, and can apply later in their own marriages. Further, one parent supports the other, enabling one to rest and providing each with a peer to consult.[19] Complementary needs exist in marriage, and the two-parent marriage provides the opportunity for one partner to complement the other.[20] A further advantage of living with two parents accrues to the children. One parent can minimize the impact of the other's irrationalities,[21] providing a safe harbor for a child during a storm. And two-parent homes, when happy, result in a collaborative approach to socializing children.[22]

Fathers serve as emotional as well as economic factors in a marriage. "By allaying the mother's anxieties, doubts, and frustrations and by making her feel competent, secure, and self-confident, the husband/father can facilitate the emergence and maintenance of responsible mother-to-child behavior."[23] Fathers "contribute to the credibility that mothers have with their children, and this may be an important factor in the mother's effectiveness."[24]

Parents can establish proper examples for children.[25] Does divorce establish improper examples? What is the child of divorce up against? When a couple divorces, their children lose a psychological support system.[26] As disciplinarians, single parents, fathers as well as mothers, "may be less controlling—and less capable of being controlling if they wanted to be—than parents who are partnered. The single-parent situation inhibits parental authoritarianism."[27] Likewise, the cooperative and consultive environment found in two-parent families disappears with divorce. The remaining parent loses someone with whom they can talk, share responsibility and compare perceptions.[28]

Children in a divorce must confront a different world. First, they have lost their models and their protectors. Gone is the support system. No longer are two parents sharing values with their offspring. In fact, no parental values are transmitted.

> As parents separate, differences tend to become accentuated and criticized. What the child perceives of his parent is thus filtered through this screen of negativity. A parent may be so anxious to pass his value systems on to a child and mitigate the value of the other parent that he pushes too hard. Such an approach leaves the child confused and likely to reject the values of both parents.[29]

Says the same researcher:

> Parental failure to help in this trying time also alienates the child from himself. The child cannot cope with the overwhelming nature of his feelings. He defends against them. He denies, represses, withdraws, regresses, projects, and detaches. He retains in fantasy what is not there in reality and he does not adequately deal with the loss.[30]

And it is quite a loss. The family represents a home base for the adolescent stepping timidly and guardedly into the world.[31] If the world presents too much turmoil, the adolescent can always return to home base to catch his breath. But the stable home base has to be there. "The need for a stable family structure is very great."[32] The adolescent needs to feel free to take the timid and guarded steps into the world. "The child needs to liberate himself, not to have it done for him."[33] The question arises, does divorce force a hasty liberation on a child, with negative results?

The child views divorce not as a problem between parents but as a threat to his security. "Even where a parent is cruel or the strains in the relationship so great that divorce would ultimately benefit him, the child has no assurance that his lot will improve. He feels betrayed. He may feel so hurt that he never trusts again. The younger the child, the less he can understand, the more his need for both parents, and the more his need for a stable family unit, the more divorce will leave him feeling betrayed, angry, hurt and untrusting."[34] One child of divorce told an author that the divorce ended her parents' fighting "but I still didn't feel peaceful inside."[35] The more messy the divorce, the more negative the impact on child development.[36] In one study, researchers found "the children experienced a parent's departure from the home as indicative of a diminished interest in them. Six- to twelve-year-old boys, as a group, felt the most rejected by their fathers, regardless of their psychological condition."[37]

Within the family, "boys without fathers reported that their mothers expressed less affection than boys with fathers did."[38] However, this can be offset by father surrogates — an uncle, grandfather, a male neighbor.[39] Still, the public perceives children of divorce differently.[40] In one study, "several women reported janitors scolding their children in a way they could not have if the children's fathers were at home."[41]

Daughters suffer, too. In one study, "daughters of divorcees were low in self-esteem," and whether missing a father through death or divorce, "both groups of father-absent girls had fewer feelings of control over their lives and [had] more anxiety than father-present girls did."[42] Also, father-absent children have difficulty delaying gratification.[43]

Some people may argue that children will not suffer in a divorce if stable contact is maintained with the absent parent. But one researcher says: "Contact weekly or every other week, of several hours together, does not provide the continuity of awareness as living within the same household."[44] Furthermore, another researcher found that five years after the divorce "only 30 percent of the children and their fathers were able to build and maintain a mutually rewarding relationship . . . ''[45]

And there are other negative factors. "Children of separated parents often feel cheated of the happy intact homes in which they imagine other children grow up."[46] Such feelings can be prolonged.

> Memories of a painful divorce can provide ambivalence in the child which festers into emotional problems in adulthood. Examples of extreme results of this deprivation can be (1) an inability or unwillingness to form lasting emotional ties with others, and (2) perpetuating the "failure syndrome" by entering into marriage, having a family and becoming divorced.[47]

Society plays a part in this. "Although prejudices seem to be declining," says one psychiatrist, "divorced parents and children suffer from their own and others' perception that their family constellation is deviant and inferior."[48] There is also the erroneous perception that once done, divorce has taken its toll never to have a negative impact again. However, the author of *Growing Up Divorced* reports that the children she interviewed responded differently depending on their age. "Each stage of development, it seems, engenders its own emotions and its own need for the separate parents, regardless of the length of time since the divorce."[49] Say two researchers: "All the adverse effects of divorce are not immediately observable. Results are sometimes not apparent until years after the event occurs."[50]

Says another scholar who has written extensively about divorce: "I would like to see a study of adults whose parents were divorced when they were children that probed their memories of the divorce and of their adjustment to it."[51] The next five chapters do just that.

ENDNOTES

1. *Marital Status and Living Arrangements: March 1981*, p. 1.
2. *Marital Status and Living Arrangements: March 1986*, p. 1.
3. Masnick and Bane, p. 21.
4. *Marital Status and Living Arrangements: March 1988*, p. 25.
5. Ibid., p. 1.
6. *Marital Status and Living Arrangements: March 1986*, p. 3.

7. Cherlin, p. 25. [This does not include separations. When they are included, two researchers say, two-thirds of all first marriages break down (Martin, Teresa Castro and Larry L. Bumpass. "Recent Trends in Marital Disruption." *Demography*, Vol. 26, No. 1, February 1989). One of my former brothers-in-law returned from his 20th class reunion in 1988 to report that one of the prizes awarded was for the person with the most divorces. It went to a woman who had been divorced four times — three of those before she was 30.]

8. Weiss, *Going It Alone. The Family Life and Social Situation of the Single Parent*, p. x.

9. *The State of Families*, p. 10.

10. *Marital Status and Living Arrangements: March 1981*, p. 1.

11. Weiss, *Going It Alone*, p. xi.

12. Cherlin, p. 81.

13. Schmid, Randolph E. Associated Press story dated April 20, 1983.

14. Blood, p. 46.

15. Sears et al., p. 79.

16. Laiken, p. 32.

17. Weiss, *Going It Alone*, p. 261.

18. Udry, p. 281.

19. Blood, p. 461.

20. Blood, pp. 38, 41.

21. Weiss, *Going It Alone*, p. 270.

22. Blood, p. 135.

23. Lewis, Michael; Feiring, Candice, and Weinraub, Marsha, "The Father as a Member of the Child's Social Network" in Lamb, *The Role of the Father in Child Development*, p. 279.

24. Hoffman, Martin L., "The Role of the Father in Moral Internalization" in Ibid., p. 375.

25. Udry, p. 181.

26. Toomin, Marjorie Kawin, "Counseling Needs of the Child of Divorce" in Cull and Hardy, p. 89.

27. Weiss, *Going It Alone*, p. 94.

28. Weiss, *Marital Separation*, p. 173.

29. Toomin in Cull and Hardy, p. 95. [Emphasis in original.]

30. Ibid., p. 90.

31. Wallerstein and Kelly, p. 82.

32. Ibid.

33. Sommerville, p. 227.

34. Toomin in Cull and Hardy, p. 92.

35. Laiken, pp. 26-27.

36. Wallerstein and Kelly, pp. 316-17.

37. Ibid., p. 48.

38. Hoffman in Lamb, *The Role of the Father in Child Development*, p. 371.

39. Biller, Henry B., "Father Absence, Divorce, and Personality Development" in Ibid., p. 490.

40. Arendell, Terry, *Mothers and Divorce: Legal, Economic, and Social Dilemmas*. Berkeley: University of California Press. 1986.

41. Weiss, *Marital Separation*, pp. 76-77.

42. Biller in Lamb, *The Role of the Father in Child Development*, p. 505.

43. Ibid., p. 517.

44. Weiss, *Marital Separation*, pp. 187-88.

45. Wallerstein and Kelly, p. 238.

46. Weiss, *Marital Separation*, p. 197.

47. Roberts, Albert R., and Roberts, Beverly J., "Divorce and the Child: A Pyrrhic Victory?" in Roberts, p. 96.

48. Lamb, Michael E., "Parental Behavior and Child Development in Nontraditional Families: an Introduction" in Lamb, *Nontraditional Families: Parenting and Child Development*, p. 6.

49. Francke, p. 14.

50. Roberts and Roberts in Roberts, p. 87.

51. Bohannan, p. 137.

Chapter Two

The Family They Remember

THE DIVORCE

What is a divorce like for the children?

Vanessa remembers her parents separating many times before they divorced when she was 14 1/2. She had a sister, 16, and a brother, 4 1/2. Vanessa, now 71, remembers an unhappy family life. "There was constant quarreling and tension between my parents, and on the children's part, fear of our father using physical violence on our mother."

Rachel, 66, an only child, has a different memory.

> I remember visiting a lawyer's office with my mother. I did not understand what it was about. I don't remember anyone explaining anything to me at any time, but I did notice a change in our living arrangements.

Rachel was seven years old. Cassie, 55, was five when her parents divorced. "Because I was so young," she says, "there was no dramatic moment."

These and many other examples speak to the uniqueness of each divorce. Tension, surprise, vagueness, violence – all are memories of family life around the time parents divorced.

However, divorce is more complex than that. It occurs in stages, according to Paul Bohannan. He writes about the six stations of divorce: (1) the emotional divorce, (2) the legal divorce, (3) the economic divorce, (4) the coparental divorce, (5) the community divorce, (6) the psychic divorce. The emotional divorce, Bohannan writes, centers around the problem of the deteriorating marriage; the legal divorce [is] based on grounds; the economic divorce . . . deals with money and property; the coparental divorce . . . deals with custody, single-parent homes, and visitation; the community divorce [involves] the changes of friends and community that every divorce experiences; and the psychic divorce [manifests] the problem of regaining individual autonomy.[1]

So while Vanessa and Rachel have different views of their respective parents' divorces, they are really revealing the station of divorce they remember best. And children of divorce, in retrospect, do not remember any station above all others. In some instances, they have suppressed their memories.

The emotional divorce is the stage that evokes the bitter memories. Jack C. Westman and David W. Cline say that even before a couple decides to divorce, they enter a period of disillusionment. "During this period," they note,

the marriage relationship is strained and the children receive the backwash, even when open conflict has not occurred. At the very least, the rift between the parents creates an atmosphere in which their children lack an image of emotional honesty between adults.[2]

Age plays a factor in how children remember and perceive their parents' divorce, although it does not neatly follow any pattern. Again, it may have to do with which station of divorce a person recalls. Nevertheless, Judith S. Wallerstein and Joan Berlin Kelly break down the age groups affected by divorce this way: preschool, 2 1/2-5; early school, 6-8; later school, 9-12; and adolescence.[3] Based on what I have learned, I would add college and adulthood. Even those age groups feel the impact of their parents' divorce, although in ways not yet fully studied.[4]

Larry recalls nothing. He was 4 1/2 and suddenly living with his grandmother. He found out about the divorce when he heard his grandmother, uncles, and aunts talking about it. Billie was eight years old when her parents divorced, yet she has little memory of the event. Anne, two years old at the time of her parents' divorce, says she did not realize her parents had divorced until she was a teenager.

> I must have known when I was much younger, but no one ever mentioned it. The subject of my father was completely ignored in the household. My father died when I was 10, so before that time I did not even know of his existence. As a teen, I became very upset and jealous of the fact that all of my friends had fathers and I had none. I used to imagine how it would be to have a father of my own.

Research suggests that the younger the children, the greater the impact of a divorce. The 3-6 age group is the one most affected, and it is between these ages that a child's personality is molded and his attitude toward marriage is formed.[5]

Alice endured much. "My mother left four times and divorced my father twice," Alice, now 41, recalls.

> The first divorce occurred when I was five. She returned when I was eight with a new baby with many health problems. My father remarried her and adopted the baby and nursed him back to health and she left a year later to live with the baby's dad.

The most difficult parting occurred when Alice was 17. "One of the neighbors, my friend from school's parents, saw my parents' divorce and my mother's marriage license [in the newspaper] — same section, same day — to the guy she lived with for eight years. I was embarrassed."

Age has an impact on how children perceive their role in a divorce. Younger children, for example, do not feel responsible for their parents' divorce. Older children often do. And older children are more likely to carry fears of abandonment and betrayal into future adult relationships.[6]

Mildred, for example, always expected her father to return and restore the marriage — a typical reconciliation fantasy among children of divorce. Her parents separated when she was three weeks old and she recalls hoping for six years that all would become right.

> I only saw my father once a week or so when he came by the house to leave the child support payment. I looked forward to his brief visits and would keep a vigil on the front porch until he came. I would count the cars as they went by, hope the next one would be his. I was terribly disappointed if he didn't come. There was no reconciliation.

Maureen's mother left in a rage one day, shoving Maureen (age five) and her sisters (seven and nine) out the door with her. "I felt strange, cheated, weird, different," Maureen says. "I reverted to wetting the bed, thumb sucking and stammering and my grades were a disaster. I was removed from a safe, sane environment into one of disordered chaos with no money, no food, no furniture, no security."

Tammy, at age five with two younger sisters, says: "I don't remember being unhappy, but I remember being a bit frightened." Edward, at 17, had a different reaction when his parents divorced. "I was stunned. I felt I had been betrayed. Divorce was still considered somewhat scandalous in those days [1960s], and I felt like the victim of an accident. I had become one of them." George, 15 years old when told by his mother, broke down and cried. His brother, 17, aware of the deteriorating marriage, reacted with a lack of concern which further confused George. George had no idea his parents' marriage was falling apart.

Lydia was eight years old when her parents divorced. She recalls the scene:

> We were walking home from a movie down a hill. They began arguing, and the next thing I knew, my father went up the hill and my mother and I went down the hill to our apartment. That was the last time I recollect them being together as my parents. I will never forget the picture in my mind of that night. It was bewilderment. Running from one to the other trying to get them to walk together again. I remember very little about my early childhood. It's as if I have blocked it out. Only the really

good and really bad incidents stand out in my mind. The day-to-day living pattern is gone.

Regardless of a child's age, the actions of parents affect their children, and parents can scar their children's psyche.[7] In Pauline's house, a civil war ensued. She remembers a fight between her parents and a frying pan flying across the room and almost hitting her younger brother. "We're going to Aunt Marjorie's for the weekend," Pauline's mother said to her husband. "You be gone when we get back." And he was.

Pauline's brother was deeply affected. He was close to his father and felt the impact of his father's departure, Pauline, then 11, says. "My brother was difficult to live with. I started taking over the household work and took care of my brother (not very well at first). My brother sided with Dad and I sided with Mom. The divorce was like the Civil War."

For Anna, the emotional scar is different. "I cannot remember being hugged by either of my parents," she says. "I can't remember anything I liked about my mother. I always wanted to be away from her. She was not kind or caring." Anna was 10 and living with her mother and brother.

And still another different reaction: "I found out about the divorce from my mother," recalls Harriet, then 13. "I was, in a way, happy, at least to see the fighting end. I wasn't really surprised. From what had been going on, I knew it was inevitable."

Generally, children start with a positive base for home life. "The image of the archetypal parents and of the home is inherent in every individual, having been laid down in the unconscious part of the psyche through the experience of generation after generation," Esther Harding writes. "But in addition, as we know full well, these images are modified by the personal experience each one has had of his personal home and parents."[8] Harding refers to the experience of children from broken homes as "faulty and most unfortunate, with far-reaching consequences for their psychic development."[9]

Jim, then 11, grew up during the Depression in a family that displayed no affection. He and his younger brother knew that their parents' marriage was deteriorating. Jim's mother was unfaithful with more than one man and eventually Jim's father became aware of this. "I felt helplessness, rejection and rage, all muted by my awareness of a non-working marriage," Jim says. At the same time, he says of his mother:

> She was a good homemaker, a light disciplinarian, probably deficient in this thing we now call nurturing. She demanded and got good housekeeping habits from her two sons. She taught me to read recipes, bake and cook in a basic sort of way.

A lack of awareness of marital infidelity also prevailed in Jill's house. She was eight. "Father was rarely around. Mother cried much of the time. Lots of secrets I would sometimes stumble onto, like a picture of him with his girlfriend. Conversations ending abruptly when I entered a room."

In Bob's house, life was just the opposite. His parents owned a small motel in Florida and he recalls life as normal and happy. One day his mother said the motel was having problems. She and Bob and his only brother (9 1/2) moved to Baltimore to live with their grandparents. Bob's father stayed behind for a year. When he moved, he moved not to Baltimore but to Washington, D.C., where the family had lived before going to Florida. Only later did Bob become aware of the divorce, and he is not sure today at what point his parents agreed on it. In Florida? After his mother moved? Did she spirit the boys out of Florida on the pretext of a visit to the grandparents? He does not know.

The divorce of Leroy's parents similarly caught him and his older sister unawares. "There was no tension, arguments or any overt signs of a split," he says. His parents called a family meeting and announced the divorce to 10-year-old Leroy and his sister. "We were devastated simply because we had no inkling."

Leroy was not really devastated by the divorce, though. What really affected him and what affects many children of divorce is that they see their world destroyed. They do not worry about the inadequacies of their parents' relationship with each other, Bohannan says.[10] Instead, children concern themselves with their relationships with both parents. As long as those relationships work, the children's world is intact. In a divorce, Bohannan says, "children mourn what they see as the passing of the family.'' Only when children have been through horrible situations are they willing to approve their parents' divorce.

And that does happen many times, usually when the father drinks heavily and/or physically abuses at least one member of the family. In Kristen's case, her father frequently beat her mother and once abused both her and one of her sisters. Twenty-three years later, Kristen speaks for many in the same circumstance when she says: ''I felt the divorce was the very best answer to a terrifying situation.''

Marjorie Kawin Toomin says that to cope with the complex set of emotions brought on by divorce, a child might detach emotionally. ''A child can seldom deal with this complex of intense feelings alone. He needs parental support to allow their full expression as well as to gain tolerance for ambivalent feelings.''[11]

Another scar that divorce inflicts on children is their feeling that they caused the divorce. As Westman and Cline put it:

> Because of their immaturity and natural tendency to see the world only through their own eyes, children generally exaggerate their own roles in causing the divorce. Frequently the cost of supporting children and the general burdens of raising children are reasons husbands give for leaving home. In addition, arguments between parents often revolve around the misbehavior and management of children. There ordinarily are many ''proofs,'' such as these, in the minds of children that they are, in fact, the villains causing the divorce. Furthermore, children understandably feel that the departing parent is rejecting or abandoning them, perhaps, because they have not been ''good'' sons or daughters.[12]

Diane feels that way. She was four years old when her parents divorced and is now 35, married for 15 years, and the mother of two children, ages 14 and 10. She spent part of her younger life in a boarding home. ''I think that perhaps I always felt we kids were put away because we interfered with our parents' marriage.'' But that scar has a positive side. ''That will not happen to my children,'' she says. ''They are loved and wanted by both of us, even though we may fall out of love with each other. Children are not pawns to be used in the game. They are thinking, feeling people.''

A parent can convey to a child the feeling that the divorce is his fault. Margaret remembers her father physically abusing her mother and her. What remains with Margaret today, at age 59, is her father's drunken refrain: ''You're not my daughter.''

Margaret overcame the taunts, in part, because she never loved her father. She recognized that he was an alcoholic, and his abusive treatment of her widened the gulf between daughter and father. ''He never showed any affection or interest in me at all,'' she recalls.

A different type of impact comes from parental silence, when neither parent will explain the divorce. It means children must invent explanations.[13] It was not unusual for respondents to my questionnaire to report they did not know why their parents had divorced. Some would say they suspected one cause when the divorce took place, but learned differently as the years went by. Others were never told anything and had to piece together the reason or reasons in later years. Mike, a 29-year-old documentary film editor in California, says that when his parents ended their 17-year marriage, he and his brother were assured an eventual explanation when they could understand the matter better. They have not received it. And even with parents still living, few children have the courage to approach them decades later to ask why.

Some form of trauma can occur during the breakup of a marriage.[14] Harold, then 12, was whisked away from school by his mother in the middle of a class.

> She was in her apron and in tears. We were carried away to seclusion in a police car. It was extremely traumatic and my first knowledge of home trouble. Things had blown up at home that morning and mother came to school to get me. We were locked out of our own house and had to get police help to even get back to get a change of clothes, my schoolbooks and personal things.

A few weeks later he learned about the divorce, including matters of his custody status, on the front page of his local newspaper.

Gloria was 10 when her parents divorced. So shocked was she by the event that she denied it, as she had unconsciously denied events leading up to it. For Gloria, the divorce caused depression. "For a few years I would tell myself I would wake up and find it a bad dream."

Louise recalls the fights. Her father would come home drunk and her parents would fight. Once her mother pulled a knife on her father and her father retaliated by breaking her nose. Louise was 12. "My brother and I had many sleepless nights." Today, though, she views the divorce not as bad but as good. "In one way the divorce was a relief because there would be no more fighting."

Beth's father, an Indiana state trooper, chose a gun. "Sometimes when he was angry, he would get his gun, put bullets in it, and twirl the barrel. Then he'd leave, usually for the shooting range. I always gave him credit for leaving." Beth was 12. She had a brother, 13, and twin sisters, seven years old.

Other anxieties arise. When the break occurs, children at first fear for the loss of their family. Then they become concerned about the remaining parent's suffering, depression, and physical health.[15] Janet first suffered as her father endured bankruptcy then unemployment. Odd job after odd job did not ease her anxiety. One day he left. Janet was 11, had just graduated from elementary school, and was looking forward to attending junior high school with friends. The anxiety grew. "Mother was angry and upset. She had no money. We were left penniless, the rent wasn't paid, and all the furniture, linens, dishes were in storage. I was frightened by my mother's reactions, and I was very hurt by my father's action."

Martha was eight years old. When Christmas arrived and her father, a traveling salesman, was not at home, she knew the family had broken up. She tried not to cry, but eventually suffered through nightmares and bed wetting for five years. Sara E. Bonkowski reports that the intensity of divorce-related questions does not decrease as the length of time after a divorce increases.[16] The anxiety also continues.

Acrimony between parents can rub off on the children in unexpected ways. It serves to alienate the children from both parents.[17] This is what happened to Patricia, who was 19 when her parents finally divorced. Her mother drank and her father escaped. "My

father made me angry because he always left me with my mother,''
Patricia recalls.

Fed up with both parents, she precipitated the divorce.

> It was New Year's Eve and my mother had been drinking
> heavily. My father left her at a party and came home. She
> came later. He had barricaded himself in the spare bedroom
> and she tried to burn down the door. I called the police.

Her mother left the state and the divorce followed.

Divorce can have another result. Wallerstein and Kelly say that a
child can cope and make sense of a divorce when

> he understands the divorce as a serious and carefully consid-
> ered remedy for an important problem, when the divorce ap-
> pears purposeful and rationally undertaken, and indeed suc-
> ceeds in bringing relief and a happier outcome for one or both
> parents.[18]

Robert S. Weiss argues that while parental separation is critically
important to the children, "in the long run, it will be only one of
many determinants of their well-being and is likely to be out-
weighed by the others taken together."[19]

That was Cindy's immediate reaction. She was 12 years old and
one of seven children. Twenty years later, she recalls:

> The morning after my father left, my mother called us all into
> her room and told us she had asked him to leave and was going
> to file for divorce. My first thought was that I hadn't had a
> chance to say goodbye, but it didn't really seem to matter. I
> never saw much of him anyway. Then I went down and made
> Mom some coffee.

Paulette, now 36, says "As a 10-year-old, I think I saw it as a
kind of adventure that would all work out fine in the end." Donn,
then six years old and now 47, says that many things happened
when his parents divorced—he moved and he lost his dogs, most of
his toys, and his family. "The divorce was one trauma in many and
was hardly noticed." Such reactions are the exception, not the rule.

RELATIONSHIPS

Divorce affects the way children perceive their parents.[20] "I thought my mother was weak," says Jill, who was eight years old when her parents divorced. "She cried easily and often. She covered for him when he drank and lied and I knew it. My father confused me. He didn't know how to have a conversation of any depth with me. I studied my friends' fathers and I knew how it should be."

Jill was so affected by her parents' negative role models that she developed a counter-model. Now 46 and a school teacher in California, Jill talks about raising her son. "When he was an infant, I talked to him and respected his opinions. I always prepared him for new experiences by talking to him about what was going to happen." Jill also made sure her son received affection as well as attention.

> When I was four or five, I saw my parents kissing just inside the bathroom door. I wanted to join them, but true to character, my father slammed the door in my face. Now, if Craig sees Gene and me hugging, we open our arms and say "Family hug," and all three of us have a three-way hug and kiss.

Howie compensated a different way. His father, a post-World War II soldier, left when Howie was three years old. "My earliest memory is one in which my father is saying goodbye," he says. Lacking a father, he created one. "I fantasized what my father was like and created an image and presence to provide some rudimentary balance to my life."

Divorce also realigns relationships.[21] Grant, then 10, first developed a father-son relationship with his grandfather. And when his mother remarried, "I had a real genuine dad, who I loved and still do." Theresa, four years old, had a different experience with her grandfather—one of stress and tension; "he never had time for me." She didn't fare any better with her grandmother, who took care of Theresa and her younger brother while their mother worked. "She fed us and made sure we behaved. I don't ever remember being showered with hugs and kisses."

Cassie's experience was just the opposite.

My grandmother and I were very close. My grandmother was the real mother figure in my life. My mother, I've since realized, became the father figure. She went off to work each day and I looked forward, as a child, to her return at suppertime. My grandmother, though, was the true nurturer, the constant in my life.

And Vanessa was happy with both grandparents. She recalls that her maternal grandfather was very loving and tolerant. Her maternal grandmother

was top banana. She ruled the roost with a firm, gentle, loving hand. I never heard my grandparents disagree on anything. Every time my parents separated and we went back to live with her, she always welcomed us with open, loving arms. With her, there was always room for one more.

The relationships that change the most dramatically are those with the absent parent and that parent's relatives. The effect is long term, if not permanent.[22] Billie, whose parents divorced when she was eight years old, did not see her father again until she was 19. "So I felt a longing and loneliness in my heart when other girls talked about their dads. I envied them the sweet, easy relationships they had and the way their dads would hug them. I desperately wanted to call someone 'Dad.'" Further, she could not get affection from her father's side of the family. "I wasn't allowed to see my dad's family and they are very warm people. In fact, that's the hurtingest separation of all. My dad's people really loved us and showed it. We'd have had lots of fun growing up near them. I regret the loss," says Billie, now 51.

One relationship that counts more than others regarding children's well-being immediately following a divorce is the one between mother and child.[23] Mothers become an important source of support to their children. Catherine expresses a refrain found in the responses to my questionnaire: "I felt my mother loved me. I remember her as gentle and kind. Even at three it bothered me that she would go hungry so I could eat. In spite of our lack of material things, my mother made me feel secure at this time in my life. I loved her."

Parental love, Blood says, "helps to create an adult who can trust and accept others. . . . One who feels loved is able to love another."[24] Thus, the long-term influence of loving relationships that existed before a divorce can extend beyond the trauma of a divorce. Bob, who was 11 when his parents divorced, remembers a good relationship with his father.

> I worshipped my father as a role model and best friend. Every weekend of my life we seemed to have fun — playgrounds, museums, parks, movies, horseback riding, go-kart tracks, boat rides, fishing, stock car races. I was aware my whole life of having more fun with my father than most of my friends had with theirs. All my life my friends enjoyed my father, who had a genuine gift for entertaining and enjoying children. He died when I was 21, of complications of alcoholism.

Today, at 33 and the father of three, Bob says: "I consciously try to be exactly like my father and to exactly recreate my happy childhood for my children. I think I largely succeed. We go to the same places, do the same things, and the kids love it all." Bob is an example of research findings that suggest a boy becomes a man (and by implication, a father) when he has a pleasant childhood and he and his father have a good warm and close relationship.[25]

Other research suggests that children of divorce perceive their relationships with their father or mother less positively than do children from intact homes.[26] As simple as that truth might sound, especially when applied to the parent who left the family, respondents to the questionnaire tended to have the same feelings toward a parent after the divorce as before. Take Ella, for example. "I don't ever recall liking my mother very much. She often took sides and punished me. My little sister lied a lot. My mother made a big deal about my sister's curly hair and paid to take her to a beauty shop, then sent me alone to a barber shop." At 68, Ella continues to feel the same way about her mother. She believes that her mother's relationship with Ella's children was the same as it had been with her. "She disliked my daughter. Preferred my sister's nine children. They were all raised in a manner she could identify with. Mine were like me."

The lasting bad feeling that comes from divorce can continue through a lifetime. Roberta, 39, twice married and once divorced, says: "I believe that I developed a wariness and cynicism about lasting relationships. I never took love for granted. I had less respect for my parents." Samantha, now 28 and divorced, says: "The divorce had a very bad effect on my life to this day. I felt I wasn't wanted by my mother, and my father hardly ever came around because of her. My life today is still so confused and mixed up that sometimes I get so depressed I just cry, and because of how I feel I try and explain everything to both my children. Sometimes I'm jealous of my friends because they have a good relationship with their mother."

Some children rise above the divorce; others do not. "Every child is not a hero," Harding says, "and not everyone has the courage to undertake the struggle for freedom voluntarily, while for others the problem is complicated by unusual disturbances in the image of the father and even more disastrously in the image of the mother that they have experienced in their personal lives."[27]

ENDNOTES

1. Bohannan in Laswell, Marcia E., and Laswell, Thomas E., eds., Love, Marriage, Family, Glenview, Illinois: Scott, Foresman and Company, 1973, p. 475.

2. Westman and Cline in Ibid, p. 465.

3. Wallerstein and Kelly, p. 312.

4. One such study recently reported is Barbara S. Cain, "Parental Divorce During College Years" in Psychiatry, Vol. 52, No. 2, 1989, pp. 135-46.

5. Roberts and Roberts in Roberts, p. 86.

6. Bridgewater, p. 9.

7. Harding, p. 134.

8. Ibid., p. 17.

9. Ibid., p. 16.

10. Bohannan, pp. 106-07.

11. Toomin in Cull and Hardy, p. 104.

12. Westman and Cline in Laswell, p. 467.

13. Bonkowski et al., p. 44.

14. Leslie, p. 553.

15. Wallerstein and Kelly, p. 47.

16. Bonkowski et al., p. 43.

17. White et al., p. 15.

18. Wallerstein and Kelly, p. 17.
19. Weiss, *Marital Separation*, p. 223.
20. Toomin in Cull and Hardy, p. 101.
21. Westman and Cline in Laswell, p. 465.
22. Fine et al., p. 710.
23. Ahrons and Bowman, p. 66.
24. Blood, p. 109.
25. Udry, p. 71.
26. Fine et al., p. 707.
27. Harding, p. 122.

Chapter Three

Life After the Divorce

FRIENDS

The impact of divorce extends beyond disrupting the child's world of parents and grandparents. Also altered, even severed, are relationships with friends. One immediate explanation: When adults divorce, one parent (usually the mother) and the children move to another neighborhood or town. Benjamin Schlesinger found that 40 percent of his subjects had moved to a new neighborhood after divorce and that this resulted in changes in schools and friendships.[1] Even when the child remains in his neighborhood, changes in relationships with friends can take place.

The outward change occurs when the parent retaining custody moves. "I lost all of my friends," Theresa recalls, "because we moved out of the neighborhood." In her case, four-year-old Theresa, her mother, and younger brother moved out of their apartment and she received no explanation about the divorce until she was 16.

Jim, whose parents divorced when he was 11, says he had no continuing childhood friends. And no wonder. After his parents divorced, he attended six different schools in grades four through nine. Paulette recalls attending 12 grade schools in six years — three in the first grade alone. "We moved from place to place so often that I never had a chance to cement a relationship with other kids. When I entered a new school, I inevitably gravitated to the underdogs."

Friendships break up for other reasons. For instance, parents sometimes forbid their children to associate with children of divorce, although the reasons vary.

In some cases, it is because of the divorce. Nellie, now 22, was raised in a family that relied on the church for both religion and education. She believes that this is what happened to her. "All my friends at church were gone because their parents wouldn't let them associate with us," she recalls 11 years after her parents divorced. "I experienced the same at school. Attending a private church-funded school, I felt like everyone thought I was weird or dirty because of my parents."

Harriet, also 22, reports a similar experience. She was 13. "I went to Catholic grade school and most of the girls I hung around with weren't allowed to see me anymore. I guess anyone whose parents were divorced wasn't good enough for their kids."

In other instances, parents forbid relationships because they do not want their children playing with children who lack parental supervision.[2] In some cases, a custodial mother works all day and leaves her children at home to play in the neighborhood. Harriet again:

> Most adults in our neighborhood (not all) treated us like we were no good. We had no parental supervision and we ran around all the time. I guess I can't really blame them for their attitudes. I pretty much stayed away from adults when I could. It seemed like they always kept an eye on us, since my mother didn't take real good care of us.

Muriel had a similar experience. Since her mother did not get home until 5 p.m., she was not allowed to have friends over after school. The restrictions extended to overnight visits. Muriel was 10 at the time and self-conscious to the point of shyness because of a missing parent.

Everyone suffers anxiety in divorce, both the parents and the children. Divorce makes everyone feel vulnerable.[3] Ruth represents an extreme case. When her parents divorced, she was sent to an orphanage without explanation. She was six years old. John, who was two years old when his parents divorced, had to learn to accept the situation. He did that in part by lying, telling his friends in grade school that his father was dead. He continued telling that story in high school.

Meg, 13, made up a different story.

> The divorce made me feel uncomfortable and I denied it in my mind by always telling any new people my dad was in the

service overseas. The way it bothered me the most is that it made me feel as though I wasn't quite as good as my peers.

Another 13-year-old also used World War II overseas service as an explanation for her father's absence. She did it because she hoped for reconciliation. A father returning from war provides a pat explanation for his prolonged absence and, in fact, gives it heroic dimensions. Sylvia's anxieties came out in a different way. She says she grew to hate her friends because they had parents. "I felt cheated of a normal family life," she says, "and resented my friends for having one." Sylvia was 14.

Life's relationships are intertwined. Child-parent relationships are important, but they are not independent of other relationships, such as peer group relationships.[4] Karen made up for the loss of her parental relationship by leaning on her friends. She was seven years old and able to overcome the move to a new neighborhood. She quickly made new friends. "Two of these friends are still very close and we have maintained a sister-like relationship for over 35 years," she says. Anna, too, relied on friends but in a different way. "I watched my friends closely and patterned myself and my life after them," she recalls. "Thank God, they were a nice group of people. It probably saved me from some really bad mistakes." Anna was 10.

Marian was two or three years old when her parents divorced. Like Karen and Anna, she made friends and learned from them. "I loved to go to my friends' homes where there was a mom, dad, brothers, and sisters, and would hint and hope for an invitation to supper." Julie, 10, behaved similarly.

> I enjoyed being around friends whose parents had a good relationship. Also, friends whose parents did things with them and invited me, I felt like they really wanted me to go, not just feeling sorry for me. Teachers at school were important to me and I tried to make a good impression on them.

Betty Lou's parents divorced for the second time when she was two years old and she did not find out who her real father was until she was 38. She recalls that her world centered on her friends.

I looked to friendships as others might look to family. I looked always for mother substitutes or sister substitutes. I really, really would have died to keep or find a best friend. I was often away from home and school was where I lived.

Other children of divorce behave in what might be considered an opposite way. A child of divorce, Ethelyn H. Klatskin says, "may unconsciously try to establish distance rather than intimacy in his peer relationships in an effort to protect himself against a potentially painful involvement."[5] "I smiled and laughed constantly in an effort to hide how rotten I felt inside," Jill recalls. "I too became an emotional cripple. I was fairly popular because I was cute and smiled a lot. Lots of superficial talk and jokes. Lots of suppressed anger. Depression and tears in privacy." Jill can trace part of her emotional problems to her mother. "My mother was bitter, hurt, angry and she generously shared her feelings with me." Ten years after the divorce, when Jill was 18, she went into psychotherapy for four years. "It worked," she says.

At first, 15-year-old George suffered from what he perceived to be a prejudice against him by his friends. That perception affected his behavior which, in turn, affected the way his friends treated him. "Though I'm sure it was mostly in my mind," he says 16 years later,

I felt my friends were uncomfortable around my house and, in a sense, had pity for me. Because of my insecure feelings, I was always trying to impress upon them that things were quite normal around my house. I never lost any friends but I think a few were driven further apart because of my feelings of being the black sheep of the group.

The loner self-image recurs. Nancy, then eight years old, says: "I felt like an outcast. Other side of the tracks (for a while). Primarily let others influence this thinking, as divorce was unacceptable status." Roseann, then seven years old, adds: "At the time I didn't realize any difference but later in my teens I found it harder to relate to other kids my own age." She describes herself as lonely but proud.

Paulette, repeatedly bounced around from school to school, says:

We were objects of wonder, and our friends' parents were unsure about allowing us to be friends with their offspring. I remember scraping plates in the cafeteria in exchange for my lunch at school and feeling proud of it until I realized that my "job" was just to make it look good. The other kids resented our being treated differently. Teachers wanted to help me with getting proper clothing and doctoring. I feel that there was a prejudice against us, but I am not sure whether it was because of our being poor or our being fatherless — perhaps both.

In some limited circumstances, children of divorce found a positive side to their parents' divorce. This was especially true in those homes where tension dominated. Half of Katherine's life was consumed by an absent, drunk, or abusive father. Her mother was unhappy. There were no family activities. Relationships with friends were thin. When her parents divorced, Katherine, then 16, could cement relationships with peers. "For the first time in eight years, I could bring my friends to my home. My mother would be cheerful instead of sad or angry or tired, and we knew my father would not come barging in to pick a fight."

MATURATION

Divorce causes immediate feelings of unhappiness in children. To the child, that seems central at the time, but Wallerstein and Kelly are concerned that the family disruption will somehow affect long-range development. They ask might divorce "slow him down in ways hard to remedy, impede or interfere with his continued development, or move him perhaps prematurely into a phase for which he is not quite ready?"[6]

It is a difficult question to answer, given the number of factors that can affect human development. In retrospect, children of divorce provide a variety of answers.

For Mary Sue, her parents' divorce when she was eight years old did affect her development. Now widowed and 62 years old, she says, "I still don't feel very mature in many ways." Mary Sue

admits that she grew up in a sheltered environment, which could
have had as much effect as the divorce. Diane thinks that may have
affected her.

> I didn't acquire any friends until grade four when I attended
> public school for the first time. Given the circumstances of a
> boarding school, I was overprotected. Logical thinking and
> questioning that come progressively through maturity didn't
> come until a few years after my own marriage. Friends (ac-
> quaintances) thought me to be strange and different. I didn't
> know how to behave like the others. I was out of touch.

On the other hand, Edward, who was about to graduate from high
school when his parents divorced, had a different experience.

> The divorce had the effect of catapulting me into adulthood. In
> some ways, growing up was easier. I did not have to grapple
> with a transition stage to maturity. I felt I was handed a raw
> deal and did not have to justify my actions to my parents. I
> would now deal with things on my own terms.

Sandra also took a somewhat jaundiced view toward life. Her
father had walked out when she was 12 and never returned. Even
her mother did not know where he had gone. "I was hostile, bitter,
self-conscious, sad, suicidal, promiscuous, sarcastic, recalcitrant,
rebellious," says Sandra, now 33. "I had to mature somewhat to
help out around home. But emotionally I really only began to mature in my twenties. My peers (What friends?) probably matured
more serenely and evenly. I tend to remember adolescence as very
rocky, sad, and troublesome."
Life at home leading up to the divorce affects children later in
life, although how is not yet known.[7] Margaret, recalling fighting,
screaming, drunkenness, and abuse, notes that her mother left home
for two weeks. "My father locked my sister and me out of the
house. All our clothes were on the porch in grocery sacks. We
stayed with an aunt and then found a furnished room. My sister
worked and I think Mother helped." This quagmire of rejection
affected her. "I tried too hard to make people like me. I never felt

the support and love of parents. I did not have the encouragement to go on to college or a career. I worked and gave my check to my mother, didn't seem to have any goals the way my friends did — other than marriage, which seemed to be my only salvation." Margaret, 59, has been married, widowed, married, and divorced.

Toomin writes that a child's adjustment to divorce can take years "during which time the dynamics need to be worked through repeatedly as the child's emotional strength and conceptual abilities mature."[8] For Jim, problems continue more than 50 years after his parents divorced. He suffers from a problem that began during his parents' emotional divorce, which occurs before the legal divorce. "I did begin stuttering and stammering about a year before my parents' divorce, and continue to do so to this day. My medical doctor keeps urging me to 'think better of yourself,' but after so long a period of time, I do not expect to overcome the problem." Jim did have a 27-year-career as an Army signal officer, but he is still nagged by his speech problem. "I am sure I could have achieved much more without my speech problems," he says today at age 65.

Not surprisingly, divorce arouses acute reactions in children. Wallerstein and Kelly have found that many children recover from these responses faster than their parents and that girls recover faster than boys.[9] Some children have help in doing this. Aura Lee is one such person. "I was self-reliant in some ways, dependent in others. I tried to develop skills such as carpentry (building rabbit pens, turkey houses), but I was emotionally dependent, needing reassurance that I was good and a worthwhile human. I withdrew in new situations to gain attention and reassurance. If my grandmother had not been a stabilizing element in my life, I feel that any chance of survival would have been limited."

Another long-term loss that accrues to children is their impaired ability to grow up in a two-gender family. Says Bohannan:

> A boy cannot become fully a man — or a girl a woman — if they model themselves only on the cues they pick up from one sex alone. A woman cannot teach a boy to be a man, or a girl a woman, without the help of men. And a man cannot either teach a boy to be a man or a girl to be a woman without the help of women.[10]

Betty Lou recognizes this.

> I guess I was very sheltered. I didn't know about evil or believe that the world could be dangerous. I was surrounded by aggressive, self-assertive, achieving women [grandmother and mother] who did not have men in their lives. There was no male influence and none seemed desired nor respected, thus I felt very good. I guess I was taught not to count on males to save me, though I didn't think about males at all at the time.

Lacking a father at home, Gary found a model.

> At the age of 10, I started work on a farm, which had a great effect on my maturity because of involvement with older men and responsibilities. From that time on, I bought my own clothes, budgeted my money for entertainment and spending. I missed all of the childhood fun—swimming, camping, goofing off. The person I worked for on the farm was a special person. I used him as a male role model. He was honest, hard working, a good husband and father. He was a substitute father at Boy Scout affairs.

In 15 years, Gary saw his biological father only three times for short periods.

What Gary compensated for was the loss of someone who would help him develop his learning ability. Norma Radin reports that through a close relationship between father and son, a father helps his son learn how to think.[11] Gary found a substitute teacher.

Wallerstein and Kelly have found that adjustment after the divorce is based on gender except among younger children. For them, the mother-child relationship determines whether or not adjustment is good.[12] Mildred, for example, always felt overprotected by her mother. As a result, she grew up with a fear of men. "I did not want to play with my friends if their fathers were around," she recalls. "If they raised their voice or spoke sharply, I was frightened." Her friends apparently knew about it, but mentioned it only once, when she was 15.

My friend called me on the phone and invited me over and all in the same breath said that her dad was going out so he wouldn't be home for a couple of hours. He was the pastor of our church and apparently recognized my problem and made a great effort to help me overcome my problem. He showed me that fathers were just people.

One research team says that maturing boys find themselves in conflict over their choice of roles. Mother represents an important adult model, but male maturity suggests behaving like a male.[13] As Lyle puts it:

There seems to have been an awful lot of lack of direction that got resolved by trial and error. When you're a young boy running around with no father to either show you or tell you what to do or how you should do it, you tend to screw up a lot, get burned, cover up and go on trying to fake until you either figure what works or what gets you in trouble. In other words, you learn the hard way and those lessons cost in pride.

Lyle, now 37, was six years old when his parents divorced. He has been married for 12 years and has two daughters.

Herman reports a similar problem, even though he was raised by his father. His mother moved out when he was seven years old, and eventually married another man. "My mother was the family disciplinarian. All I remember from birth to age 7 was punishment of one kind or another." His father worked second jobs, so Herman seldom saw him.

I was a slow maturer and had slow growth. All my friends sexually matured before I did. Lacking a mother and with a busy father, I probably spent excessive time reading and playing fantasies. I never developed adult goals.

The lack of role models in and of itself does not impede the development of mature behavior patterns. Robert Lauer notes that culture and peers play a part in helping boys learn to be male.[14] And remember the comments of previous children of divorce who consciously (and conscientiously) studied peer behavior so they would understand how to behave. Further, as Wallerstein and Kelly point out, children reorganize their intellectual and emotional coping efforts through the various developmental stages on the way to adulthood.[15]

Kristen, whose parents divorced when she was 12, first relied on one close friend. Because she had to do some domestic chores and care for two younger brothers, she survived the "giggly teenager stage" by skipping it. In high school, she found surrogate parents among her friends' parents. She also received emotional support from members of her church and from high school teachers.

Children of divorce are known for their extreme opinions and for acting on them.[16] Beth was driven to achieve. She worked part-time all during high school and financed her college education with scholarships, loans, and jobs. "For a long time," she says,

> I felt that there was something wrong with me. I thought my father had rejected me. It made me work hard to make good grades and succeed. I had to prove him wrong and make him sorry for leaving. As I look back, I realize I missed a lot of fun growing up. I'm sorry for that.

Hank is equally intense.

> My parents were divorced in the early 60s when it wasn't such a common occurrence, so many of my friends rejected me and my sister. That had a profound effect on my life. The divorce caused many financial problems. I had to spend time after school and on weekends working to earn money for my school clothes and books. In the mid-60s I became anti-social and had little respect for adult authority and had many problems dealing with teachers and the school system. I was a confused young man growing up in the 60s, influenced mostly by Bob Dylan, Mick Jagger, and the Beatles. I hated high school and I had to work if I wanted anything. I never was in trouble with the law.

Other children matured more quickly because of their parents' divorce. According to Wallerstein and Kelly,

Some youngsters increased in maturity and independence through their need to take greater responsibility, not only for themselves but also, at least temporarily, for their troubled parents. Some adolescents who appear to do well were those who from the outset had been able to maintain some distance from the parental crisis, and whose parents had permitted them to do so without intruding on them. Many of these youngsters developed a remarkable capacity to assess their parents realistically at the same time they showed them compassionate concern. This, combined with independence of spirit, appeared to augur well for their future.[17]

However, Wallerstein and Kelly do not yet know with certainty if they are correct. They are studying children in the process of coping with their parents' divorce. Meanwhile respondents to my questionnaire provide a retrospective view of how they handled the role of greater responsibility brought on by divorce.

Consider Larry. He went to live with his grandmother when he was 4 1/2. She owned a general store. It was the Depression.

I had to make my own way. I had to make spending money. I got my own rural paper routes, covering 22 miles on a bike (for 44 cents!). From 6 years old on, I would pick potatoes or strawberries and raspberries after school. From 11 years old on, I worked in a hay field. I always had a job and would get hired back season after season.

Now 58 and married for 32 years, Larry owns an insurance agency in Michigan. He and his wife have three children.

Consider Pauline. Her parents divorced when she was 11.

There was no coal, no food, no money. Mom got a job as a salesperson. I became a survivor and independent. I grew up quicker. I had to make my own decisions. I had more responsibility. I could wash, iron, clean, sew, cook, manage a household, make my own way by the time I graduated. It helped me later in life, but at that time I would have traded it for Mom and Dad and home and being normal.

Pauline is 57 and has been married for 36 years. She and her husband have three children.

Consider June. She was four years old when her parents divorced. She had two brothers and three sisters.

> I remember wanting my mother to be proud of me so that it would be one less thing she'd have to worry about. I had a lot of responsibility. For the most part, I was the oldest girl living at home. My two older sisters are 10 and eight years older than me so they didn't have too long to go before they were on their own. Sometimes I was a shoulder for my mother to lean on. My mother developed a drinking habit when I was young. Though many times I wasn't successful, I tried very hard to shelter the other children from that. I saw things and heard things that I thought I wasn't old enough to handle. It didn't matter what I felt because I had to do what was necessary at the time. It was a very difficult childhood.

June and her husband have been married for nine years. She is 28. They have two children.

Donna, one of six children, endured a divorce when she was eight years old. She put the best light on it she could. "I was different because I had responsibilities – cleaning, canning, cooking. Really, I was luckier than most because I felt needed and useful."

The maturation process for children of divorce cannot be generalized. Some feel as though they matured more quickly than others. Some feel as though they matured but in ways they are not sure they liked. Others rebelled. While growing up, children of divorce also endured – for better or worse – the influence of other adults outside the immediate family.

SUPPORT SYSTEMS

Parents are not the only adults in a child's life. Just as the relationship between parents and child has some effect on the children, so too does the one between other adults and the children. In some instances, these adults become substitute parents (or at least role models) for the divorced child. Substitute parents can provide the

love and parental nurturing that a child needs.[18] Aunts, uncles,
school teachers, adult friends, and institutions in the community –
all can function in positive (or negative) ways in the life of a child
of divorce.

"Teachers were always good role models," Herman says. "My
aunts and uncles opened their homes for frequent visits. One aunt
took the three of us on trips to zoos, museums, Indian powwows,
races (midget and Indy car), carnivals, circus. She had only one
child, three years older than me. Eventually she adopted my younger brother." Herman talks glowingly of his ties to his many aunts
and uncles, summing up this way: "Visits, dinners, and picnics
were often."

Keri speaks happily of family friends providing support.

> They would take us on excursions. Two English brothers who
> rented rooms in our house were adults for my brothers. They
> were Boy Scouts as well, which helped. I was a Girl Scout for
> a while. My mother's brother, a bachelor at the time, was
> always a favorite. Even after he married and had a child of his
> own, he maintained a great interest in us visiting, renting a car
> to take the whole family to the beach or on great picnic gather-
> ings – all this including the orphan cousin we had at home. My
> uncle has always been very special to all of us. His death five
> years ago at 86 affected me quite deeply, much more than my
> father's death. Even on his deathbed my uncle was concerned
> that perhaps he hadn't done enough.

Mary Sue reports similar experiences. "The fathers of two of my
best friends eventually offered to send me on to college. My friends
and their parents were real class. I was accepted in their homes
warmly and matter-of-factly."

Children who especially need support systems, by the way, are
the disruptive children. "They are assuredly not the majority of the
youngsters who experience the divorce of their parents," Wallerstein and Kelly emphasize, "but they represented one group of children desperately in need of a supportive network soon after the
separation, both in the school setting and in the community."[19]

The quality of the support system a child of divorce leans on is important. Some support systems made up of relatives may not be the best. "Kin, by virtue of their special status and the emotional investment they may have in the marriage, may react to the separation or divorce situation in a way which would hinder, rather than help, adjustment," Graham B. Spanier and Sandra Hanson report.[20] "Apparently, the interaction and especially the support which kin offer may be tempered by evaluation, disapproval, criticism, and other intrusions which they feel free to voice."

Sandra has bitter memories of her relatives. Now 33, she was 12 when her parents divorced. She says her father associated with "very dishonest, well-known con men." As for her mother's sisters and brothers:

> My aunts and uncles (for the most part) were and are a clan of highly self-righteous southern Baptists. They made me feel like a poor, trashy, little waif. I had no relationship with the crude and ill-mannered aunts and uncles on my Dad's side. I had a senior English teacher I admired. I mostly resented adults as screwed up, dishonest cheats, and hypocrites.

Muriel, now 65, is also cynical.

> Some adults were truly kind without showing pity. Others were very nosey and faked interest to find out details concerning our family. This was difficult as we'd been raised to be respectful to our elders, but we didn't like being questioned. I think it developed in all of us, my mother included, a good "shit detector." We learned to spot phonies early on.

Laurel, 35, also has bad feelings about some of her relatives.

> I'd say about half my aunts and uncles were like my grandmother—putting us down because my parents were getting a divorce and putting my mother down also. I remember a lot of trouble with aunts and uncles and cousins who couldn't realize that we were going through a bad time and offer their support.

Laurel's brother Daniel, 36, remembers most adults as distant and impersonal.

Another account comes from Susan. She was eight years old

when her parents divorced. Today, she is 47 and separated from her third husband. Her first two marriages ended in divorce. She describes her father as a womanizer and gambler. He owned a pool hall in the small town she grew up in.

I felt I was always odd man out in every situation — from my grandfather's nasty put-downs to teachers in school. My aunts and uncles only tolerated us; neighbors didn't like my mother or us. We were treated like outcasts. Partly, I believe because we were raised in a very small town where everyone knew what everyone was thinking and doing. My mother was looked down on because she went to bars at night. This was a complete turnaround from the way she had been when my father was with us. She changed. Our whole life changed after the divorce.

When all the aunts and uncles got together at my grandparents' home on the 4th of July, it was "tear us apart" time. Everything we did or said, every move we made, was criticized. Then it was our mother's turn. Then my father's. Between bites of homemade ice cream, we were pulverized. I will always remember their looks of disdain, of contempt. I really longed to be accepted by them — and loved. I never was. To this day I blame them for all the things they could have done to help us — but didn't.

"What does your father do for a living?" a teacher would ask, and I would wish I could sink through the floor. All around me the other children would be boasting of what professions their father held. My father made another woman pregnant, he deserted his family, my mother worked in a cafe and went to bars at night. How can you brag about that?

Marian also had problems with teachers. "I remember in school that almost all of my teachers knew that my parents were divorced and they felt this was not normal at all." And Naomi: "There were a couple of teachers who reacted crudely to Mother's non-attendance at daytime school affairs and thought I was being uncooperative in not wanting to participate when the class made Father's Day gifts."

And the church can send the wrong message to a young person.

Just before her parents divorced, Glenda's paternal grandmother found a church she wanted 10-year-old Glenda to attend. "I went about a year and was taking classes to join the church at the time of the divorce. I was told I was no longer acceptable as a member by one of the 'under ministers.' That pretty well ended my church-going."

Some people would say that societal attitudes toward divorce have changed. For example, two researchers who surveyed people born in the early 1900s say that these people "can be characterized as having an orientation which does not favor divorce. A divorce in the family may be a traumatic, even disgracing, event."[21] Popular belief aside, I would suggest that such an attitude extended into the 1960s.

One change that has taken place, though, is in the role of the extended family. Robert Thamm points out that the early American family, because of its many adults, provided a support base for children if one or both parents left, died, or rejected the children.[22]

> The children had easy access to other adults who were willing to care for them and assume the roles of their parents. Because of the larger size of the family clan, a great deal of security for the children was built into the structure itself.

Rather than limit the phenomenon to a single period in time, when discussing divorce it may be better to look at the extended family as a structure that is independent of the period. Jean's parents divorced when she was four years old and again at 13. She is now 42. She has positive memories of an extended family that supported her during the 1950s and beyond. "I was very close to my two aunts and uncles my whole life," she recalls.

> One never had children and the other had three, but we were a very close family. I knew I could count on them for anything. They made me feel special. I relied on them for support when my mom worked. My uncle (with no children) is 90 now and we are still close, though 400 miles apart.

Although rare, extended family support can cut across the chasm brought on by divorce. Esther reports that her father's sisters and brothers remained faithful and close to her mother and her. "They

were ashamed of my father, I think." Her father was a Presbyterian
minister who, at age 36, left his wife for his younger secretary.

Jack, whose parents divorced when he was 19 months old, remembers the generosity of his grandparents and his aunts and uncles. "Most of my aunts and uncles were kind and affectionate. I
had several who treated me with extra care." Jack, now 55, recalls
living with his grandparents at one point and later with aunts and
uncles when he and his mother and sister were on relief.

When Martha's parents divorced in 1941, she was eight years
old. She, her mother, and her brother moved in with their maternal
grandmother and an aunt. As Martha grew up, the family support
system got larger.

> Not only relatives, but my mother's friends and co-workers as
> well. They were very supportive. I wish all children had the
> care that we received. On my father's side, they kept us for a
> month in summer and bought us clothes. They loved us lots.
> On my mother's side, they looked after us after school and
> helped her financially when possible. Completely supportive.
> I loved them all and still do.

Where Martha had her mother's co-workers, Vanessa and her
sister and brother had the neighbors. "Although we didn't know it
at the time, some of our neighbors kept an eye on us when Mother
was working, ready to take care of us in an emergency. We lived in
the small town where my mother grew up and she knew just about
everybody."

Grandparents can be supportive. Wallerstein and Kelly state that
a good relationship with grandparents can help ease the pain of
divorce for children.[23] Not only do grandparents provide a roof over
a child's head, they can also leave a positive imprint for life. Anna
says,

> My grandmother was a quiet, loving, gentle woman. She
> loved me dearly and would spend hours playing cards, Scrab-
> ble, or reading with me. She made me feel special. She was
> half Cherokee and she would tell me stories about her life and
> how she felt about things — things that I carry with me to this
> day (feelings about the earth and nature and how people must

find harmony within that context as a companion and not one mastering the other).

John's recollection is mixed.

> My grandfather was an ill-tempered person and he let everyone know we were nobodies and were living in his house and eating his food. We had lost the farm and my mother was doing housekeeping for her father and mother and doing ironing on the side for money.

John's grandmother, on the other hand, provided a positive atmosphere for the two-year-old child of divorce.

Boys need to imitate men to develop positive personality characteristics. That is where fathers come in, but what happens when the father is absent? As should now be evident, boys can learn positive male characteristics from a male other than their father.[24] Look at the number of times a man has mentioned the beneficial role an uncle or a teacher or a pastor or a neighbor had on his development as a male and the happy memories. "My uncles were very good," Larry says. "They took us swimming, to baseball games, picnics, and shows. They took me hunting and fishing and taught me trapping, about tools, carpentry. They bought bats, balls, gloves, fishing rods and reels."

Blood says, "For boys in particular, fathers are indispensable."[25] Girls need fathers, too. Paulette was 10 when her parents divorced. She was the youngest of three daughters and had four younger brothers. Paulette recalls being confused. "I had no male role model after whom I could fashion a choice for a mate," she says. And when she looked to her friends' fathers, she found them gruff and standoffish. She married when she was 18 and is now 36. She admits that her husband is self-indulgent and lax with their three sons. "They aren't above asking Dad when I'm not around because they know he'll say yes and it complicates things. I worry about the male image they are forming and I try to play up Dad's (and mine) good points and teach them that 'bad' points are human." She also says "My husband is not the man I thought he was."

Young children who lack fathers usually seek the attention of older males.[26] Rachel, whose father and mother divorced in the

1920s when she was seven years old, recalls an example of this need for male attention.

> When I was eight or nine, my mother boarded me out to a couple on a farm for a couple of weeks. The man was in his thirties, handsome and pleasant. I overheard the wife and another woman criticizing at length the fact that I had wanted to sit next to him at dinner. After that, I knew I should not make any friendly overtures to men.

And this is how Susan recalls the lack of a father.

> A little friend once told me (in referring to a mutual friend), 'Her father never did any more for her than yours did for you!' I became very defensive and started defending my father. I was very humiliated and embarrassed, even though I knew what she said was true. I envied girls with fathers. A father took you places and teased you and brought things for you. He was always there to take your part. But mine never was.
>
> I used to wish my father would come back. He did, once, with a girlfriend. He stayed 30 minutes. My mother always threatened to have him picked up and thrown into jail if he came near us children. He wouldn't support us. But I really didn't want him back—what I wanted was a father, something he wasn't.

Another relationship that can come apart in divorce is the one with parents, brothers, and sisters of the parent who left home. Diane, four years old at the time of her parents' divorce, lived for five years in a boarding school. She then returned to live in the same town as her paternal family, but she had little contact.

> In later years, when I would meet them on the street as a teenager, they were always (and I was) smiling and friendly. Sometimes it was embarrassing to pass them by and not recognize them until someone made the initial introduction. I always apologized for not knowing them. How was I to know?

And so the support system, when its members wish, can help diminish the negative impact of divorce. When its members do not wish, the result can be an unhappy childhood and scars that continue into adulthood. In divorce, the sins of the parents are sometimes visited on the children. Unfortunately for children of divorce, they do not figure this out until they grow up.

SELF-IMAGE

Remember Jim, the boy who began stuttering as his parents' marriage deteriorated, and the advice his doctor gave him in his adult years: "Think better of yourself"? Therein lies a typically negative aspect of divorce — what the child thinks of himself afterward. That self-image is something children live with for the rest of their lives or fight hard to overcome. One respondent referred to her parents' divorce as "a badge of shame which I had to wear" and added: "I had to work hard to prove I was a nice girl."

What are some of the problems divorce can lead to for a child? According to John W. Santrock and Richard A. Warshak: regression, depression, feelings of anxiety and helplessness, and lowered self-esteem. These are factors, the researchers say, that inhibit the child from developing socially and intellectually.[27]

Janet was very unhappy as a child and began to lie. "In school when I first said my father was not living at home, a teacher's expression caused me to lie in the future. I began to write 'deceased' whenever it said 'Father's name' on any form. I felt different. Everyone I knew had a normal home with a mother and a father."

Tina also suffered but for a different reason. She spent many of her years living with her grandmother while her parents lived in a city 30 miles away. The divorce meant that Tina, 11, could pick the parent she wanted to live with. She chose her mother even though they were not close. Her father was an alcoholic.

"I always felt different," she recalls today.

You see, my parents had divorced me many years previously, so I didn't find it strange to feel so different from my peer group. These feelings were intensified after the divorce. In school I was always conscious of being on the outside, of never belonging, never fitting in. I was too smart to fit in with the other social misfits, too wild to fit in with the goody-goodies, and too poor and naive to fit in with what I perceived to be the "in" group. I had terrible feelings of inadequacy, coupled with the feeling that I was smarter than most of the other kids. I was competitive with my mother, who was beautiful (really); I resembled my father. I never belonged anywhere. I felt like a total failure, even though I got good grades. I always felt like I heard a different drummer.

Tina is now in her second marriage.

Holly was five years old when her parents divorced. Today, at 41, she has been married and is now divorced with two children. "People used to feel sorry for my sister and me," she says, "and I resented this. Even now, I hate someone feeling sorry for me because I'm divorced. A happy marriage is just plain luck." When divorce strikes (the allusion to a disease is intended), children believe they have been abandoned and feel humiliated.[28] Mabel, twice married and once divorced, remembers never trying out for school activities. "I stayed in the background always, watching the others. I tried to stay out of trouble, and I was ashamed of my family situation." Nancy, once married, once divorced, and now cohabiting, says she felt like an outcast. "I actually lost status among my peers, as divorce was looked down upon in the South—a social stigma." And Ron, who was seven at the time of the divorce, says: "I was somewhat embarrassed socially about the divorce. It seemed to make me shy. I felt that people from 'broken homes' were looked down on. I often heard that idea expressed by older people."

Wallerstein and Kelly report that unhappiness among children of divorce declines around 18 months after the divorce but rises again by the five-year anniversary.[29] Gloria reports a long-term unhappiness that began with her parents' divorce when she was 10.

I became more dependent on my mother and therefore matured slower or later than my friends. It was also the beginning of a long period of on-again off-again depression that lasted until I left home in my early 20s. I still feel at times that I have immature reactions to situations I would like to be more in control of.

Bohannan notes that one reason divorce causes bad feelings is that the person who is asked for the divorce has been deselected.[30] Children of divorce often say the same thing. "If he loved me, how could he leave?" is a question children of divorce ask. As noted earlier, they feel rejected and abandoned. In addition to the rejection, divorce interferes with the way adolescents resolve conflicts and engenders a fear that as adults they will fail in their marriages.[31]

Researchers have also found that a boy's age at the time of divorce has some impact on his self-concept. Those whose parents divorced or separated before they were five years old "seemed later to be somewhat less certain regarding their possession of traditional masculine traits than were boys who were older when their parents separated."[32] Jack, whose parents divorced when he was 19 months old, says,

> I pictured myself as being some sort of misfit in my early years (up to age 14 or so). I was very insecure, never thinking of myself as the breadwinner or man of the house. I felt trapped in a life I could not understand and had only my mother's word of how "rotten" my father was. I alternated between periods of hope and utter depression.

Jack never saw his father after the divorce. He believes that he would have had a completely different childhood with a father to look up to. Despite his childhood self-image, Jack grew up to become a successfully married husband and father of three.

What about girls?

Consider the sisters named Shirley, Angie, and Lucy. Shirley was 18 when her parents ended their marriage of 20 years.

> I felt relief to be rid of him because I was afraid of him and he made me feel bad. I worried somewhat, but not much, about how Mother would manage. I developed 32 allergies, asthma, and got raped by my high school zoology teacher. I left home 4 1/2 months after the divorce and made new friends. I immediately became sexually active, which my close friends were not. I began seeing myself as hard, cynical, worldly. I began to smoke cigarettes and occasionally drink, which none of my former friends had done.

Angie, 13 at the time, admired Shirley a great deal but did not admire Lucy. "I latched onto several male teachers at school." Lucy, 10, says that

> the approval of adults became very important. I wanted my teachers to think I was the very best in my classes, that I was special. I wanted my friends' parents to approve of me and like me, and I would like for them to have loved me and made me a part of their families. I wanted my sisters' boyfriends to like me, too.

All three sisters married, but Shirley's husband left her "for someone like his mother." Today, at 39, she says "I find myself attracted to substances that keep rage at bay."

As children, Ray and Greta suppressed their feelings. Ray was 10 and Greta nine when their parents divorced. Three decades later Ray says: "I considered myself average and did not have either an extremely positive or negative self-image." And Greta: "I stayed so busy with school activities and school work, babysitting, and bowling with adult friends, that I never allowed myself an image."

Over the long term, divorce may help self-images. "Therapists and astute observers, including many divorcees, indicate that ultimately divorce may revive feelings of self-esteem, a knowledge of one's ability to cope and survive, and can contribute to a sense of inner peace and harmony."[33] Some questionnaire respondents confirmed this about their own mothers. They write of mothers who returned to college and became professionals or who started their own business and raised the children without relying on ex-husbands for emotional or financial help. In some cases, the respondents considered this a positive part of their lives; others were less certain because it meant their mothers were seldom home.

Another factor that can improve children's self-image is remarriage of the custodial parent. In some cases, what is really improved is the family's economic condition. Still, you can feel much better about yourself on a full stomach than you can on an empty stomach. Marie, who was six years old when her parents divorced, also felt better when her mother remarried a year later. "I was just happy to have a father," she says three decades later.

Blood suggests that children of divorce are not that enthusiastic about remarriages.[34] Some children of divorce are so resentful that when asked by their mother to change their name to the stepfather's, they refuse out of loyalty to the biological father. Andrea says:

> I minded having a different last name than my mother. That was always awkward for me. When we moved, Mother asked if I wanted to change my last name to hers. I did want to in a way, but out of loyalty to my father I chose not to. Even though it embarrassed me, I never regretted that choice.

So, children of divorce deal with their self-images in various ways. Some preserve their original names; others seek adult approval; others find substitute parents. Much of what happens to a child after a divorce can influence him for life. Sometimes it is positive.

ENDNOTES

1. Schlesinger, p. 13.
2. Bohannan, p. 119.
3. Wallerstein and Kelly, p. 45.
4. Jenkins, Richard L., "Deprivation of Parental Care as a Contributor to Juvenile Delinquency" in Roberts, p. 117.
5. Klatskin, Ethelyn, "Developmental Factors" in Stuart and Abt, p. 196.
6. Wallerstein and Kelly, p. 54.
7. Pfeffer, Cynthia R., "Developmental Issues of Separation and Divorce" in Stuart and Abt, p. 24.
8. Toomin in Cull and Hardy, p. 91.
9. Wallerstein and Kelly, p. 304.
10. Bohannan in Laswell and Laswell, p. 486.
11. "The Role of the Father in Cognitive, Academic, and Intellectual Development" in Lamb, *The Role of the Father in Child Development*, p. 417.
12. Wallerstein and Kelly, p. 220.
13. Sears et al., p. 95.
14. Lauer, p. 485.
15. Wallerstein and Kelly, p. 197.
16. Thamm, p. 48.
17. Wallerstein and Kelly, p. 95.
18. LaRossa and LaRossa, p. 213.
19. Wallerstein and Kelly, p. 284.

20. Spanier and Hanson, p. 46.
21. Ibid., p. 47.
22. Thamm, p. 15.
23. Wallerstein and Kelly, p. 222.
24. Lamb in *The Role of the Father in Child Development*, p. 515.
25. Blood, p. 461.
26. Lamb in *The Role of the Father in Child Development*, pp. 498-99.
27. Santrock and Warshak, p. 114.
28. Schlesinger, p. 7.
29. Wallerstein and Kelly, p. 211.
30. Bohannan in Laswell and Laswell, p. 477.
31. Pfeffer in Stuart and Abt, p. 29. (Pfeffer is citing A. D. Sorosky's "The Psychological Effects of Divorce on Adolescents" in *Adolescence*, 12(45):123-26. 1977.)
32. Biller and Bahm, pp. 178-181.
33. Kaslow and Hyatt, p. 117.
34. Blood, p. 393.

Chapter Four

Custody

THE ECONOMIC FACTS OF LIFE

The character of life before a divorce frequently determines the deteriorated quality of life after a divorce. Marriage may be the cause of the problem. As Lenore J. Weitzman points out, marriage creates the structures by which couples live. "While most married women give priority to their family roles," she writes,

> most married men give priority to their careers. Even if both of them are in the labor force it is more likely that she will forgo further education and training while he gains additional education and on-the-job experience. As a result, her earning capacity is likely to be impaired while his is enhanced. Even in two-career families most married couples give priority to the husband's career.[1]

This structure carries over into the divorce. The woman whose career has taken second place is thrust suddenly into the role of breadwinner. Of course, the divorced mother usually cannot sustain the role.

This is how Keri remembers life after her parents divorced.

> There were many things, such as music lessons, participation in Girl Scouts and later in Rainbow Girls, which I couldn't join because my mother didn't get enough money to help pay for the necessary clothes. As we grew older, my father would go to court and have support cut, crying poor, and then take his wife on trips while we had holes in our shoes. I have not forgotten this.

Gayle, whose parents divorced three times, says: "We were poor. Mom tended bar and slept all day and was gone all night. She never kept groceries and we kids wouldn't eat much because we knew she couldn't afford much." Daniel recalls living on state aid and city food. "We lived in an apartment that was cold in the winter and hot in the summer. There never seemed to be enough money to buy even the necessities."

Vanessa felt like an underprivileged child.

> I felt poor because my mother had to work to support us when it was not yet fashionable for women to work and there was no father in the house. Mother did housework, babysitting, nursing, waitressing, sewing, nursing elderly people—whatever she could to support us. She never had to ask for welfare.

In Elizabeth's case, her father almost never paid the $40 monthly child support, except when he was drafted during World War II. During the war, the money was automatically sent to Elizabeth and her mother and life became a little easier. Her mother got a job, and at 15, Elizabeth began working after school, on holidays and on weekends. Rosemary's mother worked as a secretary "on the lowliest of academic institution salaries." "Two of my father's relatives sent me Christmas checks for new clothes."

There is no understatement as Weitzman writes:

> For most women and children, divorce means precipitous downward mobility—both economically and socially. The reduction in income brings residential moves and inferior housing, drastically diminished or nonexistent funds for recreation and leisure, and intense pressures due to inadequate time and money. Financial hardships in turn cause social dislocation and a loss of familiar networks for emotional support and social services, and intensify the psychological stress for women and children alike. On a societal level, divorce increases female and child poverty and creates an ever-widening gap between the economic well-being of divorced men, on the one hand, and their children and former wives on the other.[2]

Time and time again, respondents to my questionnaire reaffirmed Weitzman's words. Divorce usually meant poverty, economic strain, deprivation, and less variety in meals. I remember the big meal on Mondays in my house was gravy bread, an economical spinoff from the Sunday roast. Just heat the leftover gravy and pour over bread. Maybe I should count myself lucky to have eaten a roast on Sunday. Maureen recalls her childhood: "I was always cold and played games on the bed, as it was the only furniture we had. We had no food in the house and mother was always gone. We ate a lot of mayonnaise sandwiches."

Respondents also reaffirm another Weitzman observation: older women and women who have been married a long time suffer the most. Usually such women have been locked into the relationship Weitzman mentioned earlier. They have either a minor career or no career and are thus not prepared to re-enter or enter the work force. "Few of these women," Weitzman writes, "can ever hope to re-capture their loss." They cannot make up for time spent raising a family.[3] According to Arthur J. Norton and Jeanne E. Moorman, six of 10 married women now in their thirties will divorce — a record high proportion.[4] The problem identified by Weitzman will become worse.

Few families are immune from the economic deprivation brought on by divorce. Alvin L. Schorr says that three out of four poor children suffer economically because they belong either to a broken home or a large family.[5] Dana, whose parents divorced when she was two years old, says "We lived from payday to payday. We had about $2,000 a year on Mom's salary. Rent was $50 a month or less." Dana and her mother also lived with a succession of aunts and uncles. It was sometimes the only way they could get a roof over their heads. As Susan describes her life: "We lived on the brink of destitution. My mother was a cook in a small cheap hash joint."

Kristen sees her emotional deprivation stemming from economic problems. "My mother was so occupied with making a living that there wasn't much communication." Lois recalls: "Daddy never gave my mother one penny toward support. I hated him for keeping my mother pregnant and then letting her spend her adult life working to rear us."

Just for the record, not everyone reported deprivation. In some circumstances, fathers dutifully provided child support and mothers were able to find jobs. One even worked her way up from Avon saleslady to area manager. Some children worked part-time and in later years felt fulfilled because they had learned economic self-sufficiency early in life. But for most, life was difficult.

Few respondents mentioned their father's economic condition after the divorce because so few knew about their fathers after the divorce. Weitzman gives an indication of what happens economically: "On the average, divorced women and the minor children in their households experience a 73 percent decline in their standard of living in the first year after the divorce. Their former husbands, in contrast, experience a 42 percent rise in their standard of living."[6]

Even greater stress arises when the mother has no job at all.[7] Harriet recalls that her mother had difficulty holding a job because she suffered from drug and alcohol problems. The family lived on welfare. They never had much money or food. "I was, and still am, very self-conscious," Harriet says.

> Kids used to make fun of me because I didn't have any money and I always had to wear the same clothes and old beat-up shoes to school everyday. I started avoiding even going to school until I finally got some new clothes.

Working mothers suffer from a double standard. In addition to the low wages they usually receive, they are frequently perceived in a bad light by their children. Sears says that children of working mothers believe they have been rejected and that older boys show a tendency toward delinquency.[8] Children also suffer emotionally because they feel the loss of their working mother's companionship.[9] Several respondents reported that, while their mothers provided for physical needs, they never provided for emotional needs. Remember Kristen's comment about a lack of communication? She also notes that her mother never showed an interest in her activities. Or, as Pauline puts it, "Mother went from being a sweet mom to a tired mom, toughened by the business world."

While a working mother may not be good for the children, working is good for the mother, according to three researchers.

If the mother had always worked or did not begin to work until about two years after the divorce, there appeared to be no deleterious effects on the children. If mothers began to work around the time of the separation and divorce, this was associated with a high incidence of behavior problems in children, especially in boys. It was as if the children had gone through a double loss of the mother and the father, which compounded their stress.[10]

Thus, a variety of stresses fall on the mother in a divorce. She loses economic status. If she does not work, she and her children suffer deprivation. If she does work — and there's no guarantee her income will even be adequate — her children may suffer emotional deprivation. Through divorce, she is cast into a man's world yet not allowed to participate fully.

As a team of researchers puts it,

If a couple divorces, the woman loses most of her right to the man's resources, but she also loses her personal dependence and obligations of service. She now stands in direct relationship to society as the head of her family. But a male-dominated society neither recognizes a divorced woman's right to head a family nor makes available to her, as a woman, the necessary resources. The divorced mother has exchanged direct dependence on one man for general dependence on a male-dominated society. Employers, welfare officials, lawyers, judges, politicians, school authorities, doctors, even male relatives and neighbors, set the parameters of her ability to take on successfully the role of family head.[11]

THE CUSTODIAL PARENT

In the first two or three years of a child's life, the mother provides a role model for the child; in the following two or three years, the father does.[12] Overall, though, in any kind of family, it is the mother to whom children report greater attachment.[13] Another researcher has found that parents provide different types of support depending on the child's sex. For example, Udry reports that "middle-class parents tend to be instrumentally oriented toward their same-sex children, but more emotionally supportive toward their cross-sex children.''[14]

Hollywood aside, most children of divorce live with their mothers.[15] The range of emotions that such a custody puts children through is varied. One negative refrain which children of divorce report comes from Pauline. Her parents divorced when she was 11 and she had a younger brother who was close to their father. Pauline's mother went to work as a salesperson. Pauline remembers her mother as sensitive and trying to do the right thing. "But we grew up hearing, 'Your father didn't keep you, I did.'" And when Pauline and her brother visited their father at his mother's, "We'd talk. Never about my life. Usually a rehash of their divorce, whose fault it was."

Another twisting thread that runs through custody involves the relationships between mothers and daughters and between mothers and sons. In general, daughters living with their mother have a role model while sons do not. Because they perceive their mother as an inadequate substitute for their father, sons may be more defiant and rebellious.[16] Additionally, even though her model is present, the mother's energy level may be such that she has little time for the children. The result is diminished parental care, which is typical in divorced families.[17]

Theresa, whose parents divorced when she was 16, provides a before and after comparison.

> Mom and I were close until the divorce. Mom would share little secrets with me that my father didn't want me to know, such as if he was taking me to the park after work. Mom would let me know. Every night she would tell me a bedtime story. She always had time for me no matter how busy she was.

Then the divorce. "Mom tried to show me as much love as she could. But I now realize it was hard. She tried to find time for me in the evening when she got home from work, but most of the time, she was tired."

Not every child is as understanding as Theresa. June, for example, believes her mother could have done better.

> My mother loved us and put us first most of the time. She is a good person. She felt that she did her best. I feel she could have done better and I don't have much respect for her. I do feel my mother is and always has been very immature. I feel she lacks self-discipline and motivation. From what I have seen, she doesn't do much for herself and she's always looking for someone to do the simplest task for her.

June was four years old when her parents divorced. The age of the child at the time of divorce affects both the child's development and the mother's emotional state. Depending on the child's age, divorce can result in an overwhelmed mother or an overprotective one. On the other hand, the child can become aggressively undisciplined or passive. Slightly older children see the divorce as a crisis and regress; other children become underachievers.[18]

Santrock and Warshak have found one developmental variable to be the parenting approach of the custodial parent. Authoritative custodial parenting typically produces children with higher levels of competent behavior and positive social competence. The sex of the parent does not matter.[19] One obvious reason for this is modeling. The child views the authoritarian person as in control and can reap security from that feeling.

Do not confuse authoritarian with disciplinarian. Children know the difference. And while discipline may not have made children happy, a greater problem arose when discipline was inconsistent.[20] Rachel explains her mother's discipline this way:

> Discipline was unrelated to teaching right or wrong. It was related to how much I inconvenienced my mother. Yelling, swearing, but often not telling what it was about—she could not find the scissors, perhaps.

Anna, too, complains of erratic discipline. "Sometimes wildly throwing things at me, screaming names, and sometimes dismissing events as unimportant. It had more to do with her mood than anything else." Joan also recalls a discipline that did not make sense.

Mother was strict, much too strict, without any compassion or understanding. She was very dominant. I felt she was unfair in too many different circumstances. I loved her, but I didn't like her. From her I learned all the things I didn't want to be. She changed more than anyone after her divorce — to a not-so-very nice mother. She became very paranoid and stayed that way for the rest of her life. I feel that my father's abuse to her made her that way.

One explanation for the inconsistent discipline may be that the mother feels busier and more harassed. She behaves impatiently with the child because she is more interested in immediate results than in the development of long-range character goals.[21] Diane sees her mother this way:

She disciplined us the way her mother did and the nuns — very strictly. They all expected perfection from a child. The general motto was "Shut up and do as you're told." She displayed lots of affection toward us, but she also reacted harshly to many things. She had two sides to her personality (and still does). She seemed sad, bitter, frustrated, exhausted, determined. She used to build mountains from molehills with her problems because she never learned to discuss them with anyone. Very nervous, jittery person. Tense. Depressed. Made herself physically sick over her problems. Hospitalized often.

The first year after a legal divorce, researchers say, is one of anxiety, depression, anger, rejection, and incompetence for both fathers and mothers. Those feelings are particularly amplified and prolonged for custodial mothers of sons.[22] In fact, a wife's feeling of resentment toward her divorced spouse may be reflected in her relationship with her son.[23] Jack bitterly recalls life with his mother.

She was an unusually strict and harsh disciplinarian, bordering on cruelty at times. She was extremely negative, depressed, a pessimistic downer who complained about her lot in life constantly. She never ever admitted to having a good day, a nice time, a happy moment.

Weiss says that for some individuals, marriage defines the person's worth. "When their marriages end they feel that they have lost more than just a part of themselves; they feel they have lost themselves almost entirely."[24]

Add to that stress, economic problems and the loss of a partner's support, and you can understand what a deselected (Bohannan's word) person goes through. Part of an adult's loss through divorce is the buffer to help her or him contend with life's difficulties.[25] The custodial parent who can overcome these stresses presents a positive model for her or his children. The parent who does not, causes problems.[26]

Ruth, raised by her father, remembers how much she feared him. Raised with two brothers, she says:

> I felt so alone and had no teenage life to speak of. My father was bitter because, I felt, he raised me so my mother wouldn't have me. He didn't want the responsibility, but knew in time he had to stick it out. He was stern, stingy, and all for himself.

Ruth's attitude toward her father, regardless of the reason, is fairly typical, according to three researchers who found that children comply with fathers more than mothers.[27]

Life was so bad in Gayle's house that she eventually went to live with another family. "Mother was overbearing, jumped on me for anything and would punish me severely." She moved in with a family and did all the household chores for room and board. What a difference in Gayle's life!

> I was with a family that were not relatives and that is where I saw for the first time that there was an alternative to bickering and fighting. I saw consistency and love for the first time and learned how to accept change without divorce or severing family ties. I gained some confidence because these people appreciated what I did. I carried my share in chores and other responsibilities.

Most children of divorce, however, cannot flee a bad situation. They must endure. Roslyn endured. Her parents divorced when she was three years old. Both of them were apparently having affairs.

As she grew older, her mother constantly complained about her. Three years after the divorce, Roslyn recalls, "I used to think: 'Nobody likes me, nobody wants me, so I'll just be quiet and stay out of everyone's way so they can't hurt me.'" By then she was encountering a reaction that Weiss writes about—her mother saw Roslyn as a reminder of a mistaken relationship.[28] "My mother used to say, 'I hate you, you damned brat, you're just like your father. If I had any sense, I'd put you in a home. He didn't want you and neither do I.'"

Other divisions can also arise. Santrock and Warshak have found that boys raised by their fathers seem more healthy and competent than girls raised by their fathers.[29] They say there seems to be less friction between sons and fathers.[30]

That does not mean girls raised by their mothers do not have problems. According to Schlesinger, girls who have lost their fathers through divorce

> exhibited tension and inappropriate assertive, seductive or sometimes promiscuous behavior with male peers and adults. Divorced girls reported more conflict with their mothers than other groups; they also felt more insecure and apprehensive around male peers and adults than girls with both parents. "They reported more heterosexual activity than any other group."[31]

Such activity also seems related to the age of the girl at the time of the divorce. Remember Shirley? She was 18 when her parents divorced and both parents had lovers. Shirley left home within 4 1/2 months of the divorce. "I immediately became sexually active, which my close friends were not. I began seeing myself as hard, cynical, worldly. I began to smoke cigarettes and occasionally drink—which none of my former friends had done." One can only speculate what Shirley would have been like if her parents had divorced when she was eight years old instead of 18.

The custodial parent can also imprint their attitude toward sex on the child or children. The custodial mother who exhibits negative attitudes toward sex, love, and marriage may pass those feelings on to her children.

This may bring about a climate in which the children feel that any physical contact with their own bodies or any touching of other people's bodies is sinful, dirty, and forbidden. Threats of punishment following discovery of masturbatory activities increase guilt feelings surrounding sexual desires, and children exposed to such attitudes may adopt a philosophy of life-long rejection of sexual activity. Therefore, parents who want to avoid these harmful effects of excessive standards of sexual continence or prudishness should try to resolve their feelings of rejection of sexual needs.[32]

What else do children miss when raised by only one parent? According to Weiss, they can miss the echelon and organization of a two-parent home. In a sense, children become junior partners with the custodial parent.[33] That also means the custodial parent is more open with the children about the parent's uncertainties.[34] In some cases, as respondents noted in the section on maturation, roles are reversed and children assume the parental role. This occurs primarily in single-parent, single-child homes. Weiss notes that the effect of persistent role reversal is not known, although children do not seem bothered by ones of short duration.[35]

The single-parent child also faces more household work, either in the form of babysitting younger siblings or just routine chores.[36] Overall, the single-parent home is structured differently from the two-parent home.[37] What does this mean for the children who grow up and become parents? This issue is discussed in Chapter 5. For now, the discussion focuses on the child's relationship with the non-custodial parent, especially the pattern of visitation allowed or maintained.

VISITATION

Relationships with the departed parents are important to children of divorce. In one researcher's opinion, examining only the custodial parent household is meaningless.[38] In my study, I asked questions about visitation both soon after the divorce and then long after the divorce. Bohannan reports that changes in relationships occur mostly between children and their fathers "probably because their fathers were more likely to be the noncustodial parent."[39] He also notes that relationships between the non-custodial parent and children before the divorce tend to remain the same afterward.

Elizabeth, whose parents divorced when she was four years old, recalls visits once or twice a year.

> That routine remained most of my life. When I was older, instead of visiting me for a few minutes at home, he took me to one Broadway play (*Carousel*) and two restaurant dinners. When my children were young, he and his wife visited us for a 10-day period. Except for the visits, I never heard from him except a birthday and Christmas card and a letter when he wasn't feeling well. I later realized that his wife had done all the writing, and to the day he died, I never received a letter not complaining about a physical ailment, even something as insignificant as a cold. When I was younger, he just dropped by for a half hour to an hour and left. He gave me a 50-cent piece, had friendly conversation, and left. During the "adult" visits, he was always warm and friendly. He died last year.

Romayne says that the visitation pattern established in her household proved successful. She was eight years old at the time of the divorce.

> Basically, I saw my Dad once a week except for two years when I lived with him and his family. Then I saw my mother on weekends. My parents allowed me to set the guidelines on visitations. They had my best interests at heart. They never played one parent against the other. I felt they wished the other well. They got along well and worked out any problem that came up without going to court. It was what I wanted. My father enjoyed having me around. I was a very good child and he liked having me with him. He was just my dad and we enjoyed being together and sharing and fixing and eating our meal. We'd laugh about some of the things we made that didn't turn out.

Nancy recalls being her father's favorite. At the same time, she says, "He seemed apart from the family unit, distant, but I loved him." In the first year of the divorce, Nancy rarely saw her father and when she did, it was traumatic and tearful. In later years, the frequency of visits increased, but an air of tension always hung over the visits.

> Father would come to the door or sit out front and honk the horn for us. Sometimes it felt like he was just there to meet court requirements; other times we all had great times and felt good together. I looked forward to being with father. I still loved him no matter what had happened.

Visitation sometimes created problems for the children. Cassie recalls times when her father's visits embarrassed her.

> When I was perhaps 10, my father sometimes showed up in a car outside the school playground at lunchtime. I wanted to die! How everyone stared as I sat in the car with him for a few minutes. I only remember him visiting once following a birthday of mine. He brought a lot of small presents wrapped together in yellow cellophane: a stuffed dog, a doll. I was very uncomfortable on another birthday. He took me to a furniture store where I picked out a chair, lamp, and bookcase for my bedroom. I was miserable. He was obviously uncomfortable and I wished he would stay away.

Instead, Cassie and her father had an on-again, off-again relationship into her adult years (reported in the next chapter).

Alice lived with each parent at different times. Her relationships were the same before and after.

> When I lived with my mom I very seldom saw her. She worked nights, drank a lot. My dad, on the other hand, was always there. He worked days, slept on the couch. He was very mild mannered, had a nice sense of humor, and was compassionate. No matter who I lived with, the other parent never came to visit. When I lived with my mother she was always running away and hiding from my dad. When I lived with my dad, he would give me bus fare to go visit with my mom whenever the urge hit me. My mother always called me "trou-

ble." My dad was glad to see me, I guess. Well, he never called me "trouble" anyhow.

Dee's parents divorced when she was 14. Her father announced that her mother did not want to live in the house any more.

My mother was never demonstrative, but I wanted to hold her and have her hold me. My mother lived in an orphanage until being adopted at the age of 10. I don't think she was properly bonded in her childhood and her capacity to love was limited. She simply wanted her freedom.

Her visits with the children were inconsistent. "She used to drive around and stay in the car while we huddled around the window of the car. She stayed in the car while we talked small talk." By the way, Dee would like to ask her parents questions about the divorce, but they are both dead. Dee is now 27.

Mike, then 12, saw his father as the head of the household and the disciplinarian. But, after the divorce, Mike found a slightly changed man.

Occasionally, we would go to his apartment, often to the beach on Sundays. But if he just came over to our place, then it was mainly to sit and talk, eat ice cream and what not. He definitely wasn't strict, I think because he had such precious few hours with us that he forced himself to maintain an easy-going edge. At first I felt pity for him, but as time went by I began to realize that his personality was honed and developed to its ideal state only as a reaction to the divorce, which forced him to analyze himself and reassess his attitudes toward others. So I felt better and better for him as time progressed.

These responses seem to be the exception among the people who answered my questionnaire. Most responses fit in with Gerald Leslie's findings that, as distance from the divorce grew, so did the emotional distance between children and their non-custodial parent.[40] Quite simply, the number of visits by the non-custodial parent declined over time.

Mary Sue, now 62, recalls her father visiting three times in 10 years. As far as she was concerned, he had abandoned her. Pauline says she felt rejected, cheated, and unloved and for two years would not visit her father. "I spent my teen years trying to get even with Dad," she says.

Carol had to spend half of each holiday with her father at his house.

> There was a lot of ill feelings between us because he knew that we did not want to be there at all. I'm sure he only insisted we stay with him to get back at my mother. He would accuse us constantly of telling tales to my mother. He was right. We reported everything. I was very bitter toward him.

Gloria reports a relationship that went from good to bad.

> We spent every other weekend with Father. As time progressed, we went less and less. By the time I was 15 or so, we would only see him on holidays. The first year of visiting, we'd just go to his apartment and vegetate. Nothing really special. For a period of time around 12-13 years old, I was a great problem. I would be by myself in his bedroom all weekend watching television and living in my own world. I didn't want anything to do with him.
>
> Immediately upon being told of the divorce, I had a terrifying feeling of protectiveness toward my father. I remember sitting on the couch and saying, "I still love you, Daddy." I still felt close to him for a year or two afterward, but then my confused feelings began to change and I still don't understand why. At first I began feeling a sort of really stagnant despair and pity for what I perceived as his loneliness. Then I began to dislike him, everything about him. It turned into almost a hatred. Strong stuff. I despised him, and it even went to the point where I couldn't bring myself to touch him. Talk was useless.

Again and again, the story is the same: distance makes the heart grow colder. In many instances, visitations started on a grand scale and then trickled to nothing. In part, the visitations trickled to nothing because of the children's preference. They grew older and less interested in their non-custodial parent. Perhaps sensing that he could do nothing about the growing chasm, the non-custodial parent did little to stem the loss of interest.

Ties remain strong when the visits are weekly or even more often. In such circumstances, the child feels stronger attachment to both parents.[41] Bob, whose family moved from Florida to Baltimore, began to see his father a year after the divorce. "He visited Baltimore nearly every weekend and we boys went to Washington for a weekend visit every four to six weeks. We did the same things we did before the divorce. We always had fun; frequently we took along friends."

By contrast, Diane reports her father's fidelity to maintaining his Sunday visits.

> He generally picked us up in his car and drove us to his house. Then he sat in front of the TV with cans of beer to while away the afternoon. We would play in the backyard. He was curious and unattached. He gave us money and anything else we asked for, but didn't spend much time involved with us. Sometimes he asked about our home life with Mother and our school.

And how did Diane feel toward her father? "Curious and unattached."

Bob notwithstanding, Toomin says it is difficult for a father to provide a masculine principle in his child's life on a limited contact.[42] Wallerstein and Kelly say that when the non-custodial parent lacks legal rights to share in major decisions, many withdraw. Children see that as rejection.[43] Adult children of divorce bitterly report the diminished contact they experienced as children.

Finally, most of the talk about the need for a present father focuses on boys. Girls also need fathers in order to grow up as girls. They need fathers as models so they can achieve satisfactory heterosexual relationships.[44] However, that does not come across in the responses to my questionnaire. More typical is the respondent who overcame the disadvantage of a poor relationship with her father to become a happy spouse and mother. Norma talks about the difficulty she had and still has with her father.

My father usually came through in a real crisis but the every-day wants and needs of a child from a parent were only given in money, if at all, but never in time and of himself. Whenever I wanted to see my father, including today, I must call first and set up a time when it suits him. While I never expressed it to him, I am loaded with resentment.

The message that comes through repeatedly is one of resentment or discouragement. Time and time again, though, female children of divorce overcome these feelings. They report happy marriages despite the negative model their fathers may have provided.

PARENTAL COOPERATION

Couples can have a successful divorce — one that does minimum harm to the children, one that leaves the children feeling positive about themselves. Bohannan says that parents must resolve their own conflicts, that both must parent as soon as possible after the divorce, and that a network of friends must exist.[45] This section concentrates on the subject of parental cooperation.

As already noted, it is important for children to have a good relationship with their non-custodial parent after a divorce. Michael E. Lamb points out that this good relationship derives, in part, from the child's relationship to his mother and the mother's relationship to the child's father. If the mother engenders a good relationship, the child will have a better relationship.[46]

Martha, who saw her father only three times between 1941 and 1951, remembers her mother advising: "Be kind to your father. When he's old, he will need you." Martha's mother practiced what she advised. When Martha's father visited, "we put our best foot forward and served him a home-cooked meal. He was a big show. He wanted to impress us. He's the one who lost, not us." Today Martha says, "I know this is hard to believe, but it is true and I do believe that because Mother did not instill hate into us, it made it easier for us to adjust."

Jill's mother, on the other hand, instigated as many bad feelings as she could.

My mother was bitter, hurt, angry, and she generously shared her feelings with me. I wanted to call his girlfriend and ask her how she would feel if someone stole her daddy. Mommy thought that was a wonderful idea and helped me find the number. She giggled as I did it. He never asked me about it.

Harriet and Ella had mothers who constantly criticized their former spouses. Both report that their fathers generally refrained from saying anything in return. "When Mother sent nasty messages," Ella recalls, "he seemed outraged but did not return nasty messages. He did mention his disgust for her using children in this way." Harriet and Ella are today grateful that their fathers did not engage in a war of words through the children.

A war of words which uses the children forces them into choosing sides. This can become a continual burden. Florence Kaslow and Ralph Hyatt offer this insight:

> If both parents refrain from disparaging their ex-partner — a person they once loved and with whom they conceived their child or children — and move on to lead a full and rich life, again or for the first time, which appropriately includes the children and a positive attitude toward a good marriage, then the children are free to explore their world and have one and hopefully two parent models of how to cope successfully with life's exigencies.[47]

For Mary, the road to a loving father was doubly blocked because her father frequently told her he did not love her. When she was 10, he left and the divorce followed. Although Mary's father was an alcoholic, "Mother never talked against my father to me. She always told me to remember the good things about him. No matter what, he was still my father. She never tried to keep me from him after the divorce." Mary summered with her paternal grandparents and saw her father. "He grew to love me," she says.

Mary, who is 59, today praises her mother because of her forward-thinking attitude about Mary's father. Her father no longer drinks and he and Mary, the only child, have a good relationship.

I will always be grateful to my mother for letting me have my father. She says now that there were many times she was terrified I would want to leave her and live with him, but she never let on to me when I was a child. My advice to young divorcees today is always the same: "Do not talk against the child's father or mother." Children can see for themselves the faults of parents, but they need some admiration for this person they came from.

Donna, the second youngest of six children, recalls that her parents' relationship was not good at the time of their divorce. About four years later, when she was 12, her mother married someone else and Donna went to live with her father.

He was friendly with my step-dad and we always spent holidays together and saw each other. Any time we wanted, we could visit. My mother and father got along pretty well. Money was still a problem, but they didn't argue anymore as near as I recall, so it was more comfortable to be together.

The message of cooperation is reinforced by many academic sources[48] as well as by many respondents to the questionnaire. As June puts it, "My parents remained friendly and concerned toward each other. I never witnessed any bad feelings when they were together." Elizabeth, who felt rejected by her father, says today that she is grateful her mother did not disparage him. That would have made it more difficult for her to cope with the divorce. "In essence," Kaslow and Hyatt say, "how the divorced person behaves during the metamorphosis becomes a model for other family members in how to deal with strained interpersonal relationships and major life crises."[49] Borrowing from Bohannan, a couple needs to make clear that they are divorcing each other, not the child.[50]

Remarriage receives mixed reviews. In Vicki's case, her concern was having a different last name from her mother's and becoming an embarrassment (or so Vicki felt) to her mother. Eventually, Vicki was confirmed under her stepfather's name. Research suggests that the child of a remarried parent does not adjust socially as well as the child whose custodial parent remains single.[51]

Billie explains her feelings:

> When I was 13 my mother married again but we stayed in Grandma's house till I was 16. My stepfather was a small (not in stature), mean, very petty man. A lawyer by day and a crumb by night. He hated my brother and me, and when we moved away with him, our lives desperately changed. I ran away to get married at age 18 after knowing my husband four weeks. My brother got out two years later. We could both have charged child abuse, but in those days you just took it. I talk to him infrequently and don't really feel he's my parent.

The only event worse than divorce, it seems, is divorce after remarriage.[52] In some instances, the same couple remarries and then divorces. In others, the custodial parent marries anew and then divorces. Those children who endured more than one divorce consistently report unhappiness with a twist. "With each marriage," says Lee, a 45-year-old attorney, "there was always the hope that this would be the one that would last and finally there would be some stability in our lives." Children of more than one divorce also see themselves as more independent, living in their own orbit.

Remarriage is a stressful time for children of divorce because it destroys any hope that the parents will reconcile.[53] At the same time, however, remarriage does offer the child of divorce some potential for good. If the custodial parent is not functioning well, the child gets a stepparent, through remarriage, who fills the void.[54] Wallerstein and Kelly found that the arrival of a stepfather suggested greater security to the children. By relieving the mother of anxiety, it also made her more content. Her contentment was then reflected in her management style.[55]

A father in the house could also help the children. Marie, who does not remember her parents' divorce, describes her mother's second marriage when Marie was seven years old: "I was just happy to have a father." For Ellie, her stepfather "was always there for support. He never was pushy and didn't discipline me. I'm sure it wasn't easy for him." Today she thinks of her stepfather as her father.

Linda says,

I have never given much thought at all to my father. I grew up within his family's affection, but never saw him. He was out with another woman the night I was born, leaving my mother to give birth at home — alone. I guess I do have some deep resentment toward him, but never realized it before. But he is dead now, so why waste my energy? I would rather just go on feeling as I have — no feeling one way or the other. I had a stepfather who more than adequately filled in and was everything a girl could ask for in a father.

Many factors influence the life of a child of divorce, from how they get along with friends to their custodial parent's economic condition. In many ways, these factors affect the children when they grow up, marry, and become parents.

ENDNOTES

1. Weitzman, pp. xi-xii.
2. Ibid., p. 323.
3. Ibid., p. 330.
4. Schmid, Randolph E., "Study: Divorce to Teach Record for Women in Their 30s," Associated Press story in the *Centre Daily Times*, State College, Pennsylvania, April 5, 1986.
5. Schorr, p. 167.
6. Weitzman, p. xii.
7. Kinard, E. Milling, and Reiherz, Helen, "Marital Disruption" in *Journal of Family Issues*, Vol. 5, No. 1, March 1984, p. 109.
8. Sears et al., p. 131.
9. Schlesinger, p. 6.
10. Hetherington, E. Mavis; Cox, Martha, and Cox, Roger, "Effects of Divorce on Parents and Children" in Lamb, *The Role of the Father in Child Development*, pp. 248-49.
11. Koehn, Janet A.; Brown, Carol A., and Feldberg, Roslyn, "Divorced Mothers: The Costs and Benefits of Female Family Control" in Levinger and Moles, p. 229.
12. Sears et al., p. 7.
13. White et al., p. 19.
14. Udry, p. 352.
15. Fine et al., p. 711.
16. Ibid., p. 712.
17. Sexton et al., p. 28.
18. Klatskin in Stuart and Abt, pp. 186, 187, 188, 190-191.

19. Santrock and Warshak, p. 123.

20. Lauer, p. 485.

21. Hoffman, Martin L., "The Role of the Father in Moral Internalization" in Lamb, *The Role of the Father in Child Development*, p. 370.

22. Hetherington et al. in Lamb, p. 245.

23. Hoffman in Lamb, *The Role of the Father in Child Development*, p. 371.

24. Weiss, *Marital Separation*, p. 71.

25. Wallerstein and Kelly, p. 308.

26. Pett, Spring 1982, p. 34.

27. Hetherington et al. in Lamb, p. 258.

28. Weiss, *Going It Alone*, p. 67.

29. Santrock and Warshak, p. 121.

30. Ibid., p. 122.

31. Schlesinger, p. 8.

32. Garai, Joseph E., "Sex Education" in Stuart and Abt, p. 253.

33. Weiss, *Going It Alone*, p. 77.

34. Ibid., p. 83.

35. Ibid., p. 87.

36. Masnick and Bane, pp. 107-08.

37. Weiss, *Going It Alone*, p. 73.

38. Sprey, Jeste, "The Study of Single Parenthood: Some Methodological Considerations" in Schlesinger, p. 18.

39. Bohannan, p. 130.

40. Leslie, p. 553.

41. White et al., p. 15.

42. Toomin in Cull and Hardy, p. 99.

43. Wallerstein and Kelly, p. 310.

44. Udry, p. 381.

45. Bohannan, p. 135.

46. Lewis, Michael; Feiring, Candice, and Weinraub, Marsha, "The Father as a Member of the Child's Social Network" in Lamb, *The Role of the Father in Child Development*, p. 284.

47. Kaslow and Hyatt, p. 124.

48. Bridgewater, p. 9; Schlesinger, p. 6.

49. Kaslow and Hyatt, p. 119.

50. Bohannan, p. 484.

51. Pett, Spring 1982, p. 13.

52. Ibid., p. 35.

53. Hodges et al., p. 47.

54. Nye, p. 361.

55. Wallerstein and Kelly, p. 290.

Chapter Five

Adulthood

AS PARENTS TODAY

Now the children of divorce are adults, raising their own children and sustaining their own marital relationships. Now they have their own families and, as Bohannan says, raising children is "the ultimate purpose of the family."[1]

Some children of divorce are like Mary Sue. "I approached parenthood with deep interest and great joy." A retired public health nurse, she and her husband of 32 years had four children. She is now a widow.

Others are like Romayne.

> I am gentle, loving, caring, affectionate, easy to talk to, easy to hug and kiss. Firm, not a pushover, not afraid to say "no" when I think it is the right thing to say. Supportive of their goals and ideas. I care about their emotional as well as physical needs. I try to be the kind of mother I wish I would have had.

Romayne has been married for 17 years and has three children.

Diane fumbled a lot by using the only model she had, her childhood, as a way of raising her children. "In my earlier years of marriage I was a terrible mother," she recalls. "I tried to have my daughter (oldest child) behave just as I was made to behave. I found out that just doesn't work." Diane solved her problem by talking to other women and learning what they were doing. "I finally relaxed — body and mind. It was a change in my way of thinking and doing things. A gradual one."

According to Udry, the most important relationship is the one developed by the nuclear family. Such ties eclipse all other kinship obligations.[2] This is the approach Carol took. Her parents divorced when she was 9-10 and she spent her youth in boarding schools. She did not marry until age 32 (she is now 46) and she and her husband have two children and two stepchildren from her husband's previous two marriages. "I feel very aware of being a family. We do a lot of things as a family. Trips, meals out, shows, excursions or even school recitals, or plays we attend as a family."

Christine also stresses family. "If our children are involved in an activity, we are there, too (one or both). My parents never attended anything that we were involved in. That always bothered me. We also give a lot of verbal and physical attention."

Other children of divorce find themselves comparing their parenthood with their childhood. This is not surprising, since we spend half our lives as children or raising children.[3] Rachel makes the point this way: "I have given my daughter the one thing I lacked most as a child: attention." Anna says:

> I wanted to give everything to my children that I had not had from my parents and discovered, happily, in the process that I got more in return than I could ever give. From my husband and children I learned what love was all about. I cannot imagine (as a parent) why I was treated the way I was. I love my children dearly. They are very special.

Ella also makes comparisons between her childhood and her parenthood.

> As a parent, I was very alert to not taking sides as my mother had done between two children. I made a conscious effort to avoid my family influence. We remained in touch but I did not want my children involved in my mother's craziness.

Some parents live the childhood they never had through their children. As Beth, a 38-year-old high school English teacher in Tennessee, puts it:

I want them to have a more secure life than I did. I want them to enjoy childhood because I don't think I did. I have a tendency to want to buy toys, shoes and clothes for them more than is necessary because I remember so little. I encourage them to participate in activities such as music lessons and baseball, and I place importance on church activities.

For Larry, the 58-year-old owner of an insurance agency in Michigan, the way he and his wife raised their three children was through love and support.

I made every effort to see that they got where they wanted to go—from early events through college. I spend considerable leisure time with them, even as grown-ups. I was a teacher for them. Taught them to fish and hunt. Taught them right from wrong and respect for people's property and for people as human beings. I exposed them to all types of experiences, from summer camps, art fairs, Indian Guides, Girl Scouts, church activities, cultural activities, that I didn't have with my parents.

Many children of divorce grow up without a good role model, for example, a father or two happy parents. Some children imitate the model they have; others reject it but have no alternatives.[4] Keri was lucky, for her mother provided her and her brothers with positive reinforcement. She even discussed marriage. "She told us that the failure of her marriage was no reason for our marriage to fail." John also lacked a two-parent model, but in parenthood he chose to emphasize to his children that they had two parents and that each was valuable.

Some children of divorce feel so strongly about the kind of parents they want to be that they sacrifice socially to be with their children. For example, Robert, 44, and his wife adopted two children.

I strive to do those things as a parent I feel all parents should do. I spend time with my family in lieu of myself. We eat out as a family two or more times a week. There is no drinking in our house, no nights out with the boys, and there was no physical discipline after age 14.

Joy, who has been divorced and remarried, knows she wants to provide a good example for her children.

The most important thing I can give, which I didn't have, is a model for a close and harmonious union between a man and woman. I did not settle for less in my marriage, because I saw my parents and others do so with disastrous effect. When there is tension, I try always to confront the situation lovingly and honestly in an effort to relieve the tension and return to the essence of the relationship—that which is real and honest.

Not every parent can give every second of his waking day to his children. Lamb states that what is important between a parent and child is not the quantity of the time but the quality.[5] George, 31, worries because he is in the process of starting his own plumbing business and feels he does not give his children (3 1/2 and one years old) enough attention.

Many times I see my father's selfishness in myself. I'm in and out of my house like the wind, kissing my wife and kids as I pass. When I do stop, I do give positive attention to my children, read them books, or play games or puppets.

Jim's parents divorced when he was 12. He and his wife of 37 years raised four sons. Jim, a physician in Delaware, chose parenting over outside pursuits.

Never having had a father's love and companionship, I tried to give these to my sons as much as possible. My profession kept me away more than I wanted, but I always planned activities as a family occasion so we could all do it together. I always wanted to play golf, but I deliberately did not learn, since it would have separated me from the family.

Samantha, a single parent with a full-time job, tries to spend her time at home with her children, "talking things over with them and trying to make them understand as best as I can what's going on." Samantha is bitter about her parents' divorce and blames her mother. Samantha's marriage lasted 10 years and produced two children.

Samantha not only missed a family when she grew up, but now her two children will miss one. Yet it is the family, Lauer says, that helps children learn what it means to be a male or a female and how to behave as a parent. A family also teaches children how to relate to others.[6]

Donna has established the role of the family early in her marriage and parenthood.

> My husband and I always make a point of not arguing in front of Amy, and we don't hold back in showing affection for one another in front of her. (I never saw my parents hug or kiss that I can remember.) I find myself feeling guilty whenever I do anything that reminds me of my parents and try to avoid any such action. I tell Amy often how much Tim and I love each other and how much we love her and want us always to be together as one big happy family.

Not all women have such clear-cut ideas about their roles as mothers and wives. Richard A. Kulka and Helen Weingarten say that women who grow up in divorced homes place more importance on their roles as mothers than their roles as wives.[7]

For example, Vera, who is 44, never worked full-time when her children were growing up "because I did not want to be away from my children like my mother was. I have had to put second my own personal life goals." Mildred also focuses on her only child. "I am outwardly affectionate, understanding, too lenient and too generous materially."

Not all women respond that way. Kristen has been married for 17 years and has two children, 15 1/2 and 14. She says,

> Sometimes I see them as a burden that if I could do it over I would not take on. I have not enjoyed parenthood since my children started school. I tend to neglect doing things with both children together because they constantly argue. I find

myself placing more emphasis on being a wife than on being a mother.

Betty Lou combines both roles. She is 50 and has been married for 28 years.

When I married (even before) I believed the best thing a woman can do for her children is to love their father and the best thing a man can do for his children is to love their mother. Of course, that is the hardest part. I truly do not want my children to add the problems of divorce to all the problems of adolescence so I work at trying to love their father. I choose to stay and that affects my choices. I wanted my children to have the security of counting on us to be there like a rock.

Evelyn, on the other hand, explains very clearly why she places such an emphasis on being a mother.

It was a blow to me after I was married to have my mother tell me that my father had "tricked" her and she never wanted to have me. So I was doubly rejected. She never could understand why I wanted to have children. I wanted to feel part of a family.

ADJUSTMENTS

Children of divorce continue to adjust as they move into adulthood and especially when they become parents. According to Kulka and Weingarten, divorce affects the way people value their marital and parental roles and how they adjust to them.[8]

Frances offers insights based on 32 years of marriage to a man who was divorced when she met him and whose parents endured 50 years of an unhappy marriage. "We made an agreement," she writes,

that one of us would remain silent if there was a fight brewing and at least carry on a polite union for the children's sake. There have been periods of icy silence lasting up to six months, but the children don't remember or were unaware of these times. I have realized that it was quite often myself that I was unhappy with, rather than it being my husband's fault. There are periods of change that everyone goes through which seem to be marked by discontent and bewilderment, "What am I doing here and where am I going?" And the easiest person to lash out at is your spouse. If these periods can be weathered with understanding and compassion, a new plateau can be reached.

Parents who have divorced childhoods begin adulthood with less well-being than adults from intact childhoods, and women suffer more than men.[9] Alice comments:

I feel my parents' divorce left me very insecure as a person. I don't know how to be a wife and mother, so I played it by ear. My husband and I are a very poor example of marriage and parenthood for my children. They deserve more, but that's life.

Vanessa also recognizes that the insecurity of her childhood continued into her marriage.

My family moved 35 times from the time I was born until I was 14, when my father left for good. My husband and I decided to postpone parenthood until we could own our own home — to provide stability and continuity for our child. I did not want her to live with the anxiety I had known as a child of never knowing where she would be living from month to month, of always packing and moving. Within five years of marriage, we had bought our first home and had our one child (the month after Pearl Harbor). We lived in that house for 30 years.

Other women report either being determined to have a successful marriage or staying in a shaky marriage for the sake of the children. Vera and her husband had only two children because Vera, who was raised alone and then by various aunts and uncles, felt she could not cope with more than two. "Parenting was such a challenge to me — staying with my children in a way my parents had not done.''

When couples marry, they base their roles on preconceptions that are the residue of childhood observations of their parents.[10] Mildred remembers that she and her husband decided not to have children because they both had to work to earn a comfortable living.

> Deep down, though, my reason was that I imagined that my husband would leave. I did not fully realize this until my son was born and he cried a lot. One day during his crying marathon, I started crying too and told him if he didn't quit crying before his dad came home his dad would leave. I wondered for a moment why I said that, and then it dawned on me that this was what I have been told was the reason my dad left. Even though it was always said jokingly, it had made a great impact.

In Keri's case, both she and her husband were children of divorce. Both worked extra hard to foster a close relationship with their children. "We both felt the need for that parental bonding,'' she says.

Udry has found that a happy marriage is determined by the consistency of the husband's personality.[11] Female respondents to my questionnaire revealed that they worked to maintain their husband's consistency by ensuring his happiness. "I work a lot harder for harmony than most of my peers,'' says Anna, who is 41 and has been married for 21 years.

> If there are arguments, and of course there are, I am always more anxious to settle it quickly. I choose words carefully to avoid scars. I take the extra steps to promote family and its importance. And most of all I work to keep my relationship with my husband a good one. I see that as the base from which the rest is able to grow.

Simone is 32 and has been married for 11 years. She says: "I do not like to argue with my husband in front of our son." Elizabeth also worked on maintaining her marriage of 30 years.

I tried very hard to keep my marriage together in spite of many problems. I succeeded and I hope that too much damage wasn't done to the children in the process. I always made it a point to let them know that they were in no way the cause of any problems my husband and I had. I had to show that I could succeed and didn't have to follow in my parents' footsteps.

Researchers have also looked at how easily boys assume masculinity. They have noted that the path from boyhood to manhood is made easier if the boy has a pleasant childhood and good emotional involvement with a warm and affectionate father.[12] After divorce, such involvement is rare given that few children are able to maintain much of a relationship with their non-custodial fathers. The few who did remember their childhoods pleasantly now attempt to provide the same atmosphere for their children.

PARENTHOOD

"My parents' divorce caused such ambivalent feelings in me," says Kristen, who is 35 and has been married for 17 years.

I was glad my father was finally gone after years of separations and fights and fear. But our standard of living changed drastically. I hated him for failing to be the kind of father I wanted. I hated him more the older I got. I can now understand how he (they?) failed. Marriage and parenthood are so awesome. I didn't really have a successful role model. I only knew the kind of family life I wanted for my children—I just am unable to achieve the desired results or to allow myself to enjoy the achieving.

As Weiss puts it, "Marriages are formed on the intertwining of many separate strands: sexual intimacy, shared parenting, companionship, mutual obligation, collaboration in furnishing and maintaining a home, love."[13] In Kristen's home, her father drank and committed adultery. He was violent and frequently beat his wife. He once abused his daughters. Kristen was 12 at the time. "I felt the divorce was the very best answer to a terrifying situation."

Parents undoubtedly provide their children with their first conception of what husbands, wives, and parents are. Udry says: "A new couple brings to marriage expectations derived from different parental homes which are not necessarily very similar."[14] Thus, the question is: What role does a divorced childhood play when a child grows up and marries?

Kristen entered marriage and parenthood with ambivalent feelings. Martha, on the other hand, knew what she wanted. "I chose a stable, dependable man who gave me security both for myself and my children. He's not flamboyant but he wears well and is a great human being." Her marriage to "the great human being" has lasted 29 years and has produced two children. "I chose a husband exactly opposite to my father," Martha says.

Gloria reports that her parents' divorce has affected her attitude, not so much toward her daughter as toward her husband and her marriage. She says she wanted a loving mate who would work with her as an equal partner. "I was absolutely sure of who I was marrying," she says, "and who I loved, was loved by so that my children would have the benefit of a whole healthy family." Gloria and her husband have been married 2 1/2 years and have a 17-month-old child. They were expecting another when they filled out the questionnaire.

In some ways, two parents are important, not for their differences, but their similarities in tasks.[15] By the same token, the role each member expects the other to take can arise out of childhood experiences. How each spouse fulfills his duty can be judged subjectively. A problem can arise when one spouse violates the other's expectations.[16] Paulette admits to such problems today.

> During my teen years I believe I fashioned a warped perception of men and marriage because I had no adults after whom I could pattern my own life. I am a constant reader and I have been for many years, but the lives I read about are only fiction. My reading is escapism and I realize with my head that it's only stories, but my heart cherishes the romance, the self-confident women, the success stories.

Paulette, 36, considers her marriage of 18 years shaky but will not leave her husband.

I think I cling to the idea that things will work out because it releases me from having to do something about the situation. My brother waited 10 years to leave his wife, my sister endured 13 years of abuse before she sought divorce — perhaps because of that same Pollyanna attitude. Our parents' divorce did indeed affect our own marriages.

Shirley also sees an impact on her marriage from her parents divorce. She is 39 and self-employed. She was married for 18 years before separating. They have one daughter. "My parents represent just one more model of a failed marriage. Less security."

The lack of a model falls more heavily on males. Girls tend to think about their future role as mothers, whereas boys seldom do. Few people entering parenthood have any realistic notion of what children are like.[17] Fathers gain introspection as they age. Janet says of her brother:

When his first child reached 4 1/2 years of age (the age at which my brother was abandoned), my brother realized how deeply attached he was to his son, and the realization of what his father had done to him was much clearer because he was a parent.

Udry points out that the parental roles are stereotyped.

There are certain expectations as to how fathers should behave with respect to their children. In actual fact, there is far more variation in the behavior of fathers than there is in people's expectations of fathers. When someone is a father, his behavior is in part controlled by the fact that he knows the general role of the father. However, his actual behavior is modified by his personality, the personalities of his wife and children, his other role commitments (Does his occupation require him to travel? Is his wife an invalid?), and by pressures of daily family life.[18]

Not surprisingly, fathers interact more with their sons than their daughters. As the boys grow older, they develop a preferential relationship with their father.[19] Obviously, when not disrupted by divorce, this relationship helps the boy. Additionally, a confident parent communicates that confidence to his children, which then enables the family to function better.[20] As Edward puts it, "Parents are there to fill the emotional needs of children, not the other way around."

In Andrea's case, that didn't happen. She is now 53. Her first marriage, which produced two children, ended in divorce. Her second marriage has lasted 25 years. She and her second husband also have two children. Andrea grew up as a stepchild and while her stepfather fully accepted and loved her, he never adopted her. "I had hoped my second husband would wish to adopt my first two children but I thought, possibly wrongly, that he should initiate the idea. He never did."

What really transpired was not helpful for the oldest son. "He was rejected by his own father, detached from his stepfather, and I was unable to make up the difference to him," Andrea says. "Also, he bore the brunt of my own instability and youth at his birth. I lost his trust when he was very little; never regained it. He is, by his choice only, estranged from the family right now and was once before for 5 1/2 years."

Rachel, too, feels that for a while she was a failure. Her responses to several questions indicated that she feels less than happy about her role as wife and mother. She revealed that she had considered suicide. She summarizes her view in a sentence: "Parenthood was so much more difficult than I ever expected."

There is a suggestion that boys who grow up in divorced homes do not make the same emotional investment in parenthood as women.[21] However, responses to the questionnaire indicate that this is not so. In general, the fathers responding to the questionnaire made conscious positive decisions regarding the raising of their children.

Women are even more vocal. "I made a careful, deliberate choice in the father of my children—a number one outcome of my divorced upbringing," says Maureen.

> I do not want to subject my children to that kind of life. I am committed to being there. I am a full-time worker. I attend concerts, plays, parties, homework, bedtimes, breakfast. I have the luxury of knowing my children. I just wish the gov-

ernment made motherhood financially easier. We all do household and personal maintenance, but parenthood is a profession, the one upon which the character of our next generation
depends.

Susan responds:

The one thing I could give my children that I did not have after
my parents' divorce was a mother at home — night and day. I
never left my children with a babysitter or alone — never. My
memories of waking deep in the night to a dark and motherless
home have never left me. I made sure I was always there.

Katherine is 46, twice married, and has five children between her
first and her second husband.

I am wonderful as a parent. I am a good role model in that I
work, I am responsible, I run a nice household, and I let them
all do whatever they are interested in doing. I am extremely
energetic and endlessly concerned, interested, and supportive
of all their doings. I realize that I am absolutely too much, and
when they make me back off from participating in their lives, I
do so. They laugh at me and think I am overbearing, which I
accept. They also love it and tell me so.
     I have consciously turned 180 degrees in participating in the
lives of my children. My parents did not know me because
they had their own problems, or perhaps because they weren't
capable of empathy. I had many substitute parents in neighbors, aunts and uncles, and teachers. I wanted to be that parent
for my children.

Other mothers do not report as much success and, unfortunately,
blame themselves. Mabel is 49 and in her second marriage. She
says she loves her children but has not been a good mother.

My oldest daughter is self-destructive (drugs, an interest in
men involved in crime). She's divorced, one child. My middle
daughter has married and divorced the same man twice. She
reminds me of my mother somewhat. She goes to a fundamen-
talist church; she has two children. My youngest is male, 25,
never married, wants to live in a kind of free lifestyle. He is a

pretty good artist. I tried to be more loving than my mother. I wanted the kids to have better clothes than I had, so I would sew at night for them. Even though I wanted to be a better parent than my mother, I am not. In fact, I guess I'm no better.

Mabel exhibits a divorced child's intense desire that somehow, some way, he or she will be a better parent than his parents. When it works, congratulations are in order. When it fails, as in Mabel's case, undeserved self-recrimination results. Divorced children as parents are always looking over their shoulders.

A QUESTION OF DIVORCE

Having experienced divorce as a child, would a person endure it again as an adult? Or, as Patricia puts it, are children of divorce doomed to divorce themselves? "How about the impact that divorce has on children when they, in turn, get married?" she asks. "Are their odds greater than children from a two-parent house to get divorced? Are their odds greater for having a larger number of spouses? To me, this is an important area: Do we really follow in our parents' footsteps?" She is divorced.

If not doomed to divorce, perhaps children of divorce see its benefits. For Darlene, 46, "divorce is an enormous blessing. Consider the alternative—to be tied unwillingly to another person. Slavery could be no more onerous." She has been divorced twice.

> Divorce has been part of my life, my mother's life, and her mother's life. It was not in any way an easy solution to marital problems, but was not the total upheaval experienced in other families, perhaps. Like diabetes, we hoped not to develop a dreaded inherited condition, but were prepared to a certain extent. I'm not sure how I made adjustments. Interestingly, however, neither of my daughters has been married, and they are well past the age at which their female ancestors married—at least the first time.

A child of divorce may consider that more is at stake in his marriage. "People often say that children from broken homes rarely succeed in their own marriages," 55-year-old Janet says. "I believe it can work the other way around. The need to prove you can succeed at something your parents failed at is a factor in many enduring marriages.'' In fact, Janet admits to such a motivation in working to keep her marriage of 34 years intact.

Blood points out that marriage means sharing in decisions and doing things together. It requires, in his words, ''careful pairing.''[22] In Linda's words,

> a person cannot be married by himself. It definitely takes two people. However, the ease of divorce and the total acceptance of the divorced state regardless of details make the success rate of a marriage understandably low. I am very pessimistic.

Linda is now separated, but her pessimism comes not from her marital experience but from her father's example.

> By now my dad has been married seven times and is our family joke. It is incredible to me that marriages fail when we are so determined to make them succeed. My dad never cared one way or the other if they succeeded, but I did. I am left with no answers or words of wisdom for my children, and that makes me feel terrible.

On the other hand, can good marriages lead to good divorces? Blood says that the central feature of modern marriages is companionship.[23] Recognizing that each person in a marriage may need a change to grow, Vera would consent to divorce. ''But I think we could part more amiably and we would both want to continue our relationships with the children. I would not want the children to experience the kind of grief I did.'' Vera, who has been married for 22 years, adds, ''But I hope we can continue to grow inside our marriage.''

Karen is less agreeable. She has been married for 22 years and has three children. Even if her husband wanted a divorce, she doubts that she would agree to one. The memories of her childhood after her parents' divorce remain with her. Her mother went from being a homemaker to a housecleaner and money was not readily available. Today, in response to the question, Karen says, ''I guess still in my mind being divorced means being alone and poor.''

Jill takes a middle view. ''At one point,'' she recalls,

I did not feel our marriage was working. I went to a psychologist/therapist. He saw us together, and Gene and I had more sessions separately. After a total of 20 sessions, Gene saw where he had to change and so did I. Now I can't imagine anything or anyone pulling us apart.

Vicky regards divorce as something she would not do—again. She was three years old when her parents divorced. Her mother was 20. Vicky is now 36 and has been married twice. Her first marriage lasted seven years; her second marriage is in its ninth year. She has a daughter, 16, and a son, three—one from each marriage.

I regret divorcing my daughter's father, but it is done. Had I had more maturity I would have tried harder to patch up the differences with him and maybe we would still be together. I do not still love him per se but perhaps we could have worked it out. This is something I will never know. But I do know this: I can work out whatever I need to with my present husband and we can stay together. We have done this in the past during crisis times. If my husband wanted a divorce, I would, after a period of time, allow it, but I would have to feel that there was no talking him out of it. What use would it be to force him to stay or not continue with his life? Should divorce happen, I seriously doubt that I would remarry for a third time.

Research over a period of nearly 20 years indicates that children of divorce are more likely to report having problems in their marriages than people who grew up in two-parent homes.[24] Thus, children of divorce such as Ruth, a 65-year-old widow, strive to maintain the two-parent home. On the question of divorce, she responds with a conditional "no." She would not divorce her husband for infidelity, as long as he showed no hostility toward the children and was not abusive.

But if he were an alcoholic, abusive, and threatening, I'd divorce him because I wouldn't want the children growing up in that environment of fear and hate. I figured that I was marked in my early years and I would not want that for them.

Pauline also feels the need for a two-parent home. She remembers her mother first as a homemaker, then a saleslady because her father did not support them. "I would never get divorced or allow my husband to get a divorce, if I could help it," she says. "I am 57, am not trained to work, and I have taken care of a home for 36 years, so I would feel I had the right to his care. I would fight divorce, even if he didn't love me. I'd be more aggressive than my mom was."

Janet says much the same thing. She explains that when she thought her marriage wasn't working, she worked to make it a success. "I didn't want to experience what my mother had been through."

Remember Frances who took a vow of silence with her husband when they were having a fight? She says this about divorce:

We are both free to be ourselves and to disagree, but respect the other. It has taken a lot of conscious work to reach this point. I know so many who have divorced and regret it, or who have remarried and found themselves in the same unhappy situation. My advice to someone contemplating divorce would be to try to change yourself and your situation within the marriage before trying to change your spouse.

Marnie, 31, has been married for nine years and has three children, ages five, two, and one. She agrees with Frances.

When I feel my marriage is not working, we discuss it, pray about it, and do our best to better it. It has always worked in the past and I trust it will continue to do so. I must say that in the first years I was probably quicker to give up because of my background. I don't seem to have that problem any more.

Clearly, many respondents remember their one-parent childhoods and vow that they will not raise their children in such an environment. To some extent, Weiss supports that feeling.

I would not agree with those who claim it is always better for
children to be members of a happy one-parent home than an
unhappy two-parent home. It is possible for individuals to be
unhappily married and yet function well as parents.[25]

He qualifies that position this way:

But if conflicts between the parents absorb so much of their
energy that they have little left to give to the children, if the
efforts of one parent to support and direct the children are
systematically frustrated by the contradictory effects of the
other, if angry quarrels keep the home in constant turmoil — if
the parents' marriage is so bad that the parents are totally preoccupied by their troubles with each other, or so depressed that
they cannot attend to their children — then the children as well
as the parents are likely to benefit from parental separation.[26]

Tammy feels her childhood was one of turmoil and was determined to have a stable home for her husband and two children. She
draws on her youthful experience "to better know what to do and
what not to do." But that does not mean not getting divorced. "A
messy marriage," she says, "would be a worse environment to
raise children in than a divorced one. If I were to divorce my husband, I would try to maintain a civil relationship with him so we
could continue raising our children."

A similar view comes from Harriet and Dick. Both are in their
early twenties and grew up in divorced homes. They have been
married for three years and have three children. They would un-
dergo divorce themselves, although reluctantly.

Harriet:

Maybe as a last resort, because it isn't good for children to see
their parents always fighting. But I believe because both myself and my husband grew up in divorced homes, that we are
more dedicated to our marriage, and I think it would take a lot
more than simple differences to take one parent away from
their children. Neither of us wants to see our children go
through what we went through as children.

Dick:

> Yes, I would divorce, because I would rather split up peacefully and maintain a good relationship with my children and my ex-spouse. I would not want my children in an environment where us parents were always fighting (as even when we argue now we can see it affecting them even to the point where they will cry just because we are yelling at each other). If we did divorce, I would definitely try to make them understand that sometimes two people can't get along. I would rather divorce than subject them to an environment of hate, yelling, and screaming or whatever and do it in peace so that the spouse could have an opportunity to see the children when they want instead of when a judge says so.

In the main, divorce does engender more divorce. "As previous studies have found, both male and female children of divorce are more likely than others to be divorced, perhaps because of low expectations of success in marriage and consequent low commitment to and investment in it."[27] Two other researchers say,

> People's experience with marital dissolution, either as involved parties or as the children of divorced parents, may lead to negative attitudes toward marriage. Among the divorced, the experience of an unhappy marriage may lead to the rejection of the institution of marriage as well as of the particular spouse. Children who live through a divorce may question the value of marriage for themselves or may, at least, be cautious about a marital commitment. Alternatively, prior experience with divorce could result in a less careful marital choice if divorce is seen as an acceptable solution for an unhappy marriage.[28]

Kulka and Weingarten, citing the work of others, add,

> A consistent though modest finding documented in the literature on marital instability is that children from parental marriages dissolved by divorce or separation are more likely than children from intact parental homes to dissolve their own marriages voluntarily.[29]

Take Ella, for example. She is 59 and a medical secretary in Pennsylvania.

> I have been through two divorces. I would hesitate getting married again. I feel that my marriage problems were mainly caused by the wrong choice of husband. I always picked someone who was an underdog. I also wasn't mature enough to handle the first marriage and always took my problems to my mother and father, who sided with me and eventually encouraged me to get a divorce. I always felt that my first husband would leave me for someone else. Today he is a fine person who made something of his life with a very good job, and he wasn't the type who would walk out on a marriage. But I was so unsure of myself that I thought he would. Most of my friends are still married and seem to be fairly happy.
>
> The second time I got married, I was afraid of being alone and unmarried. I do not feel that way anymore. I feel that, except for financial problems, I can handle my life alone. I feel that it is more important to be alone than to be married just for the sake of being married. Both my children encouraged me to get my second divorce because they knew that I was mentally and physically upset and that none of us could handle the type of mental abuse that we were being subjected to. This time, I decided for myself and feel that I have never made a better decision.

For 51-year-old Adelaide, the circumstances were different, but the result, divorce, was the same.

> I always believed that being a child of divorce, that I'd never get a divorce myself. I never even considered the possibilities. Yet when my children had left home I realized my husband and I were strangers, living in the same house but with nothing in common but our two children. Our goals in life were different, our interests and friends and outlooks were different. I had grown up and he hadn't. I had to decide, as my father had, had the past 20-plus years been all that great? Did I want to spend another 20-plus years doing the same thing, striving so hard to make a connection with someone who essentially isn't

there? The answers came back "no." Fortunately, I am able to support myself at a much higher income level than my mother was and I still have a good, non-adversarial relationship with my former husband. There is still a feeling of being a family between the four of us, but it's very fragile.

Tina is in her second marriage, which has lasted 6 1/2 years, so far. Her first marriage, which she entered when she was 18, lasted for 12 years and produced three children, now ages 24, 23, and 20. "Most marriages don't work," she says.

> They are simply a way of life. If there is no pain and you can be friends, why throw away the way of life that you have built together? I have a great deal of personal freedom, and I am able to do most of the things I want to. I no longer have the unreal expectations that some man will complete and fulfill my life. Only I can do that, and I will continue as I am, unless he makes me uncomfortable enough that I want to get rid of him.
>
> Him get rid of me? You've got to be kidding. I'm number four. He couldn't handle another failure.

For some who make up the second generation of divorce, though, a different attitude prevails. Many times those who are divorced made it a point to divorce on friendly terms and to maintain a good relationship with their spouse afterward. If not, they at least made sure their children maintained a good relationship.

Joan, now in her second marriage, recalls what happened after her parents divorced and how it affected her when she divorced.

> I saw a drastic change in my mother after her divorce and then I myself changed after my divorce. The change in my mother's personality had a great deal of effect on me, more than the divorce itself. Enough of a change for me to remember that after I was divorced, I tried to resume a natural environment so that my children wouldn't be affected. I always saw to it that they kept in close touch with their father and they still do, even after 12 years of divorce from him. I felt they need to know that their father always cared about them.

Finally, there are those who would divorce if they felt they could. Wanda, 53, has been married for 26 years. She says she would divorce

> especially if we didn't have such a stupid legal system relative to divorce and children. Also, husbands and wives themselves are often mistreated in divorce hearings and settlements.
>
> I am a very firm believer in divorces, especially with first marriages. I think the process should be handled in some sort of method other than by the usual cold, straitlaced, legal method now used. Seems that procedure just makes bad matters worse and is ofttimes mostly a shouting match between two lawyers. I believe people who have any children and then divorce definitely should not be allowed to remarry until the children are grown.

THE DIVORCED GRANDPARENTS

A couple's divorce has a longer ranging impact than might first be imagined. Naturally, it affects the children of the marriage. And when those children grow up and become parents, the divorce will have some impact on the children's children.

In some cases, such as Karen's, her children had no grandparents. In Jim's case, because he "lost" his grandparents through divorce, he made sure his sons had as much contact as possible with their grandparents. This meant the boys saw Jim's mother and stepfather. "They enjoyed visiting each other and sometimes my mother would take them on trips," Jim recalls. "We did not live close together, so visits were only several times per year. The grandparents both died when the boys were still quite young."

When there is contact with grandparents, it is usually with the maternal grandparents.[30] This naturally results from the high number of mothers who have served as custodial parents; they encourage a closeness with their own side of the family.

Recall the circumstances under which some children of divorce are raised, with the mother struggling to maintain a household and hold down a job. She has little time for her children. Pauline reports that her mother made up for what she had to miss with her children by bestowing an extra dose of love on her grandchildren — Pauline's children.

Janet reports a similar closeness between grandmother and grandchildren.

> Their relationship with my mother is extraordinary. She is admired and loved by them, and is a loving and caring grandmother to them. She has her own personal relationship with them, apart from mine, and will fly from New York to Washington to visit the older one completely on her own. (She is 82.)

Esther says: "My children were very close to my mother and spent summers with her. They were with her at home two days before she died a painful cancer death a year ago and they helped me care for her. She was so special in their lives. She helped me when they were babies. They loved her so much."

Complications can arise when couples remarry and grandchildren have "extra" grandparents. As Harriet explains it, her children are close to both her parents, although "my mother gets upset because my kids call my father's second wife 'Grandma.'"

In the main, divorced grandparents do not have stereotypical relationships with grandchildren. Even though Louise's daughter sees her grandfather occasionally, she really hardly knows him.

> She doesn't love him like a child to their grandparents. She knows who he is, but doesn't quite know how to react to him. Sometimes she'll go in her room and continue playing and ignore him. My daughter and mother love each other dearly. I feel my daughter misses some things I see other children have with their grandparents. I think she misses the closeness and sometimes material things other grandparents provide.

Jan's son has no relationship with his grandfather. He does know his grandmother, who has been married four times. He learned about the divorce when he was nine years old. "I just explained that she had trouble choosing and living with men. My son says: 'It's kind of scary to know that I have so many grandfathers without knowing them or much about them. But I don't think about it very much.'''

Margaret's children have no contact with their divorced grandparents. "When all of the children were young, they missed going to Grandma's as other kids did. At graduations and weddings, the lack of family attendance was noted."

Billie offers a similar assessment.

> My children have never seen my mother. She lived in another state and didn't even express an interest in them. My dad is unconcerned, too. They've seen him about four times. They missed out on the joys of having loving grandparents.

Connie takes a different view.

> A hard part for me is when you have to have both parents at family functions. When my children's birthday parties come up, I get very nervous just thinking about it. It's very uncomfortable being in the same room with both of them—uncomfortable for me and, I think, for everyone else at the party. Another thing is you can never talk to one parent about the other. They just don't want to hear it. It's very hard not being close to your parents. I know my relationship with them died a long time ago.

Lonnie recalls a similar fear. She was worried that her divorced, hostile parents and their new spouses would all visit her at the same time in the hospital after her first child's birth. The crisis never came because her father died before her first child was born.

Relationships with grandparents obviously don't fit patterns. Jean, who endured two divorces as a child, describes the relationships as complicated. She says:

> My children are very close to their (step) grandfather and his fifth wife. We all love him. He still drinks and knows the children don't want to be around him then. My oldest daughter visits and corresponds with my natural father and his wife. My other three children don't. My mother was very close to all of my children until her death in 1976.

Maureen interprets the relationships this way:

> My children love my father (now 82) and go bowling with him
> and treat him to Chinese dinners when he comes to town. My
> mother isn't involved with my children except to give them
> gifts. She seldom visits (and the children request that she leave
> when she does). I actually think the divorce has made my chil-
> dren richer — each grandparent comes alone and interacts with
> the children instead of catering to one another and the whims
> of age.

For Alma's only daughter, visits with Grandma were rare because she lived in Florida and Alma lived in Massachusetts. When
the two got together, however, "they had the relationship that my
mother and I never had." There is no relationship with Alma's
father. He lives five minutes away, but his second wife rebuffs
attempts at family ties. Alma's father did not even attend the funeral
of Alma's other daughter.

Finally, some children of divorce choose Holly's approach.

> I told my children my father was dead. He might as well be. I
> feel bad that they are growing up without a grandfather (my
> ex-husband's father died many years ago), but at least they
> have a father who takes an interest in them.

EFFORTS AT RECONCILIATION

When a couple divorces, many relationships end. Children are
removed from one parent or the other. Visitation by the non-custodial parent dwindles (if it existed at all). By the time children of
divorce are parents themselves, they seldom see their non-custodial
parent. Divorce seems to sever all ties forever.

In limited cases, though, children of divorce and their non-custodial parent reconcile or try to reconcile. The results are mixed.

Cassie had an on-again, off-again relationship with her father. He
divorced Cassie's mother when Cassie was five years old. When
she was 10, he would occasionally show up at Cassie's school play-
ground around lunchtime.

My father really wasn't the least bit interested in me, so far as I can tell, until I became an attractive teenager. We all lived in the same town, my father with his second wife. I used to pass his place of business sometimes and when I discovered he enjoyed showing me off to business friends, I used that knowledge to manipulate him into giving me money for prom gowns, etc. After I graduated from high school, he paid for two more years of education (Katharine Gibbs School, New York City) and even bought me a fur coat. He gave me away when I was married (leaving his wife home at my request) — (what a brat I was!) and paid for my reception. He lavished gifts on our first child at birth.

Cassie is now 55 and the mother of five children. As for her father,

We haven't seen him now for 23 years, although he used to send the family a generous Christmas check and call a couple of times a year. The last time I saw him, I tried to talk to him about the divorce and how I thought it had affected me. He was the picture of injured innocence, couldn't understand what I was talking about. We never talked of it again, and to this day I've never been able to discuss the divorce with my mother.

My father became a very successful businessman and later ran for Congress (defeated). About ten years ago, he and his wife became Jehovah's Witnesses. Now he or I write about every 18 months; my letter a catalogue of ages, births, marriages, schooling, employment. His are brief, mostly about his preaching and proselytizing.

Years ago, when he was rich, I used to fantasize that he would die, leave me buckets of money (which he had assured me he would) and I, in perfect poetic justice, would give it all to my mother to ease her Social Security years. Well, it didn't happen and somehow I think if there's any money left, it will go to Jehovah. Can it be that he is atoning?

During the 35 years following the divorce of Esther's parents, she saw her father only three times. "It was like talking to a stranger. We had nothing in common. Once I drove 300 miles to visit him so he could see my children; he wouldn't even let me come out to his house.'' Instead, they met briefly at Esther's motel.

> I think deep down I began to hate him more. Why couldn't he have been there to see me graduate from high school? Or college? Why couldn't he have given me away when I married? Or stand with us when our first child was christened?

Esther doesn't have the answers to those questions. But she has something else.

> I'm happy to report that in the past few years my relationship with my father has been restored. It happened only after I accepted Jesus as Lord of my life, not just my Savior, and I forgave my father. I wrote to my father and a correspondence followed. Five years passed before I saw him. He came to visit us for two days.
>
> As he was about to climb into our car for the trip taking him back to my sister's, I couldn't resist the urge to reach out my arms and squeeze him. I hugged him but a moment, as a child clutches a treasured teddy. His voice broke as he looked fully into my watering eyes. "How could you love me? After all I've done?" I think he knew that I had turned all my hate and bitterness over to Jesus. I think he knew that I loved because I had forgiven.
>
> God has restored my heart to my father and his to mine — and his relationship has been healed with at least three of his children. Whatever his faults, mistakes of the past, he is still my dad. God has given me a new heart to love him with.

Three years after Darlene's parents divorced, she saw her father for the first time.

> When I became engaged at 17, he took an interest and accepted my husband-to-be at a time when my mother totally rejected him. By that time, I'd had a year of college and we were thinking of leaving town. For the first time, he talked to me, an engaged woman, as one adult to another, not offering

unasked-for advice nor trying to discourage my plans. I was surprised by this reversal, but grateful for his belated support.

My dad and I have achieved a certain measure of resolution. The hatred that I once felt toward him has abated and now we can at least respect one another, even if we'll never be easy in each other's company. We exchange letters regularly, and he once apologized to me for all his parental shortcomings. The phrase "to understand all is to forgive all" comes to mind. I understand much and am still working on forgiveness.

Naomi was only 6 months old when her parents divorced. It would be 30 years until they reconciled. Her father attempted to maintain contact, but Naomi's mother forbade visits and returned all letters and packages unopened. As an adult, Naomi finally met her father.

At the moment of our reunion (I was 32, he was 58), an ocean wave of rejection washed over me—my husband had to keep the conversation going for the first 24 hours. Something deeply buried surfaced and knocked me over. Imagine my surprise when I found that many of my interests and drives were reflections of his: needlework, music, theater, books. I see my father's selfishness and do not wish to emulate it.

For Naomi, relationships changed.

My mother's second marriage coupled her to a person with whom no one in the world can get along, not even mother. In search of peace in the house, she has carbon copied his negative attitudes and judgments—and there went the darling mother of my youth. My father's second marriage hitched him to a delightful woman of character and strength who has shown me and my family nothing but sweet kindness since the fateful day we met. Isn't life wild?

Jim's parents divorced when he was 12 and he did not see his father for a decade.

Then he visited me in college. It was a hurried, strained visit, not very satisfactory. We didn't do anything but talk and we had little in common to talk about. I had gotten into church activities and was abstinent. My father visited while somewhat under alcoholic influence. It wasn't a good meeting. He was uncomfortable with me. He waited until shortly before train time to visit, so he was under stress to get away. We had little to talk about.

I was pleased that he finally made the contact with me, but I was sad that we had so little in common and that he had been willing to wait so long to see his only child. I was also hurt that he waited until the last minute to visit, so that we couldn't have a relaxed visit. All in all, my thought was, "I certainly don't mean much to my father. This is just a gesture."

In his later years, my father and I had a reconciliation, which lasted until his death. We had both changed considerably over the years, mellowing toward each other, and it was a beautiful thing to experience. It came about almost miraculously through a surprising intermediary and was a joyful experience after all those years of separation. In his seventies, my father first met his only daughter-in-law and grandchildren. From then on until his death, there was a warm relationship with me and my family, which blessed all involved. I am always grateful that this reconciliation occurred.

For Paulette, the results were different.

I cannot relate to my father at all because I resent his coming back into our lives, after we've been through all those growing pains, and trying to be "Daddy." The circumstances of his life seem to me to be not enough of an excuse to just leave seven children to fend for themselves. I think he could have done something, like hold a job, but he chose not to. We do not owe him filial devotion and he is not really asking for it — he only wants to be a part of our lives. But I am too bitter, right now, to allow him to get too close. I feel as I did when I was real young: he has so many children what does he need me

for? I am not important to him except as one of his posses-
sions, and I resent that enough to withdraw from him.

Fantasy and disappointment, perhaps partners more than we realize, enter into some reconciliation attempts. Take Vicky.

I always had the feeling that my father was being kept from me
and I from him, that if he could he would take me away from
my mother and stepfather and make my life more meaningful
and love me like no one else could love me. This, in retrospect, was pure fantasy. When I was 21-22, I searched him out
and found him to be a complete stranger to me (of course!) and
not all that interested in me or my welfare. No bells rang or
music played in the background as we ran through fields of
daisy flowers to embrace. Ha, ha. He was just a man sitting in
a chair who has progressed over the years to be a source of
problems for me. He now wishes that I would take care of
him! He has never come to see me but has called (Florida to
Idaho) several times to cry on my shoulder. He tries to make
me feel that since I am his flesh and blood that I owe him my
love and devotion and that he should be able to unburden himself to me when he needs to and that I should be sympathetic to
his whining and crying. I wish now that I would have never
looked him up. He is a man of many problems, all his own
making.

Frances feels she learned from her attempted reconciliation. She
had banished her father from her life when he divorced her mother.
Frances was 16.

I refused to have anything to do with him or see him even
though he tried. I didn't want anything to do with him and was
terrified I might see him. I can't explain this, as he never did
anything to cause me to feel this way, and my mother didn't
demand it.
He seemed a stranger [he had just spent three years overseas
in World War II] and I think I wanted to run from the whole
situation. This might have been devastating to him and I think
I was ashamed of the way I acted. My father did get in touch

with me and came to visit once when I had my own young family. This enabled me to resolve my feelings. I found I didn't like him and was glad that I hadn't had to live with him during my teen years.

Lyle had a similar experience. His memories of his father, a cook, are not good.

Most of all I remember how hard he was on me when I misbehaved. He always got in a rage and whipped me with a stick or with a belt (he put fear in my life), or he would make me spell words before I could eat or send me to bed without supper. He also made me eat things and I would throw up. But I remember most when he was in a rage he broke a sailboat I had bought with money I'd saved. We did little together, but he made me feel secure and sometimes put me to bed, which I loved.

Nine years passed.

At age 15, I ran away from home just for fun and was brought back. At 16 I quit school, left home, and went to work, which I found out was not so easy. One year later I went back to school and worked two jobs to support myself and school. One of the jobs was at my father's family business, and I thought we were getting to know each other. My father got married again and gave me a room to stay in. Well, Vietnam was on and along came the draft and he would get drunk every night and argue with me about that damned war. Finally I left and we have never gotten together ever since. He got divorced from that marriage (which also has one son) and I have heard he has gotten married again. It has always made me think that a man such as him from a big extended family, a veteran, a Shriner, a conservative, etc., could be such an abuser, alcoholic, and creep. I owe him nothing. I am the man and father I am because I work at it.

When Ruth's parents divorced around her sixth year, she first went to an orphanage. She remembers her mother's visits.

She showed her love to me, brought little miscellaneous gifts that I was happy to receive, and always said that she hoped someday I could be with her. I loved her and also wished I could be with her. I fantasized about living just with her. My heart ached to see her. But she remarried, moved away, and I didn't see her for years. I lost interest in her.

Ruth is now 65 and lives in Massachusetts. She is widowed.

I was married for quite a few years when my mother returned to this area after her second marriage because her husband passed away. She chose to live with a married sister in another town. We visited often, were civil to one another. The children loved her. But something was always missing. When I asked her to live with me after I became a widow, she declined, preferring her sister. Now I started to hate her because I was her daughter and I wanted to know her, and her promise of years ago to be together was broken. Two years ago, her sister passed away and again she refused my offer, saying she has to take care of her brother-in-law, who isn't too well. I think that's not a good excuse because he has grown children responsible for him. She herself is getting senile. I hardly hear from her. I don't know her as a mother or a friend so we've drifted apart. When I got married, I never saw my father again. We were enemies and he passed away without our making up. I never had a mother, and it seems I never will. That's what divorced parents have done to me. I've came full circle — alone again with no relatives or friends.

ENDNOTES

1. Bohannan, pp. 11-12.
2. Udry, p. 376.
3. Sommerville, p. 20.
4. Blood, p. 167.
5. Lamb, Michael E., "Fathers and Child Development: An Integrative Overview" in Lamb, *The Role of the Father in Child Development*, p. 6.
6. Lauer, p. 490.
7. Kulka and Weingarten, p. 69.
8. Ibid., p. 73.

9. Glenn, p. 68.

10. Blood, p. 202.

11. Udry, p. 274.

12. Ibid., p. 71.

13. Weiss, *Marital Separation*, p. 84.

14. Udry, pp. 292-93.

15. Blood, p. 459.

16. Ibid., p. 205.

17. Udry, p. 485.

18. Ibid., p. 353.

19. Lamb, Michael E., and Goldberg, Wendy A., "The Father-Child Relationship: A Synthesis of Biological, Evolutionary, and Social Perspectives" in Hoffman et al., pp. 68-69.

20. Weiss, *Going It Alone*, p. 288.

21. Kulka and Weingarten, p. 70.

22. Blood, p. 18.

23. Blood, p. 279.

24. Kulka and Weingarten, p. 63.

25. Weiss, *Going It Alone*, pp. xii-xiv.

26. Ibid.

27. Glenn, p. 68.

28. Thornton and Freedman, p. 302.

29. Kulka and Weingarten, p. 68.

30. Schlesinger, p. 13.

Chapter Six

The Legacy of Divorce

One of the respondents to my query for children of divorce wrote:

> My side of divorce is a very positive one. I feel that I actually benefited from my parents' divorce. I think I am more independent and more mature as a result. I guess I just want someone to write a book telling parents who do divorce that their kids do have a chance to be perfectly normal.

Leaving aside the question of what "perfectly normal" means, I agree that children who grow up in divorced homes do not necessarily turn out abnormal. Nor do they become criminals, psychopaths, villains, or lousy parents. For some children, divorce liberates them from a terrible situation: their parents' lousy marriage.

"Everyone is a special case," says Katherine, "and everyone benefits when a noisy, screaming, combative, unpredictable home is transformed into a peaceful, rational one. This is what happened in my case. I had ill effects not from my parents' divorce, but from their marriage." Katherine is now 41 and in her second marriage.

Tammy also takes a positive view of her parents' divorce.

> I think I've been blessed in my life. I feel I have a healthy attitude about life and am fairly logical. I don't know if having parents who were divorced made me any different than if they hadn't been divorced. I like to be positive about what did happen, though, and say I've learned a lot by others' mistakes.

Tammy is 36 and has been married for 15 years.

She adds:

My brothers and sisters are not as fortunate as I. Both real sisters are very unhappy with their lives and families. One is going for psychological counseling. My half-brother and sister were married and divorced (not to each other). I believe the age of the child when the divorce takes place has different effects on the child. They were in their teens during my mother's second divorce from their father (who was more a father to me than my real father). I have many beautiful memories of our second family.

Pamela also views the bickering marriage as more of a problem than the peaceful divorce. "In many cases," she writes,

divorce is preferable to raising children in an atmosphere of fighting, tension, or physical and/or mental abuse. I still think two parents are best, but one caring, loving parent is still better than two miserable, unhappy people staying together for the wrong reasons. All things considered, I think I ended up with a better, fuller life with my mother and brother than I would have with my father around.

Pamela, 51, is the mother of two. She is divorced.

Holly believes that the divorce of her parents helped build her character.

As a child of divorce (at a young age), there were times when lonesomeness took over and you felt very alone in a large world and no one understood you. But I grew from that experience in a way that I became stronger. I feel I am a survivor. I have worked most of my life. After my second child was a year old, I started work again. In talking to various people and friends through the years, I went through more in just my childhood than most people experience in a lifetime. I don't share my experiences with anyone, but someday I hope to. My divorce wasn't earth-shattering, but it has left me a bit of a loner and I don't like to socialize with most people. I basically like people but don't trust anyone, which includes my family.

Holly is 41 and the mother of two. Her marriage lasted six years.

Divorce does have a negative impact. One research team has

found that divorced mothers tend to use more negative sanctions with sons than daughters. This has led the team to say: "Sons of divorced parents seemed to be having a hard time of it, and this may in part explain why . . . the adverse effects of divorce are more severe and enduring for boys than for girls."[1] Deidre S. Laiken suggests that girls are less affected because they rarely act out their feelings in antisocial ways. "We are more likely to turn the anger, the confusion, inward upon ourselves. Weight problems, insomnia, depression, anything that might be self-destructive is more acceptable for a girl and a woman."[2] One respondent to my questionnaire wrote: "There must be psychological ramifications to growing up as a child of divorce. I am a compulsive overeater, recovering with almost 20 years in Overeaters Anonymous. Directly traceable to my reactions as a child."

Norval D. Glenn supports that respondent's analysis. "We found in our much larger sample a slightly greater difference at the older ages than at the younger ones, which suggests that the negative effects [of divorce] persist undiminished throughout the lifespan."[3] Kulka and Weingarten report similar results.

> The one rather consistent difference which does emerge — a greater tendency for adults from divorced backgrounds to identify childhood or adolescence as the most unhappy time of their lives — suggests that the impact of parental divorce as a stressful event does indeed endure through one's lifetime.[4]

This is how Andrea describes the phenomenon.

> I enrolled the children of my first marriage under my current married name to spare them the embarrassment I felt at being different. So many times I had to explain the difference in my name and my mother's and that involved explaining that my parents were divorced. I found that humiliating and wanted to spare my own children that embarrassment.

Three sisters (Carla, 32, Joleen, 30, and Mary Kay, 27) compared their answers to my questionnaire and discovered that all three had been sexually molested by different men. The youngest, who grew up feeling very unloved, says,

I have had to come to terms with my childhood. I think that had my parents not divorced, I would not have been molested. My father was never around and I feel like it was a male adult telling you to do something — an authority figure. I feel that it had a profound effect on my life, not at all good, and I feel my parents' divorce was directly responsible for it happening.

Samantha also endured negative feelings.

The divorce had a very bad effect on my life to this day. I felt I wasn't wanted by my mother, and my father hardly ever came around because of her. My life today is still so confused and mixed up that sometimes I get so depressed I just cry, and because of how I feel I try and explain everything to both my children. Sometimes I'm jealous of my friends because they have a good relationship with their mother.

Samantha is 28.

Elizabeth, a 55-year-old secretary, observes:

My friends who came from unbroken homes seem to have better self-esteem and sureness in themselves as individuals, and two of the main places I see this is in their choice of mates and careers. I did not follow through on college although already enrolled; did not think I was smart enough to be an attorney, which I wanted to be. I was always attracted to men as needy as myself and never felt the acceptance and approval I always wanted from the men in my life. I have always overreacted and translated anger toward me or strong criticism as rejection.

In fact, the effect of divorce can extend beyond one's immediate generation. As Cindy, a 32-year-old single parent, explains:

My mother got a dose of man-hating from her mother. She gave me a double dose. I suppose I've given my daughter a triple dose. But just the same, she's better off as she knows that nothing's really fair and if you want something, you have to work for it. Before my parents divorced, I didn't know women didn't have to get married and have kids. I thought that's all there was. I was 18 and a parent before I really knew

I'd have to work for a living. It's a bad start she won't have to overcome.

I chose to be a single parent, not because my parents were divorced but because of how they were before. I am decidedly anti-men. I didn't want my child exposed to the fears I had as a child; coping with one parent is all any child should be asked to do.

Margaret sees the matter differently. She hasn't seen her father since she was 12. She is 59 and was married at age 19 for 10 years and widowed. She married a second time at age 32 for 23 years then divorced. Her children are 38, 34, 25, and 22.

My biggest worry now is that my grandchildren will not have a normal family life either. My goal and hope was that we would be happy grandparents and have a home for all the kids to visit. I never had parents or grandparents to look up to and I wanted that for my children. I realize the world and morals are much different now and divorce is widely accepted. My grandchildren will surely have many friends in the same circumstances.

*   *   *

What can be said about the children of divorce who participated in this work? What themes dominate, especially in their lives as parents?

If one were to check through the responses to see how frequently words appear, one word that would rank high is *over-protective*. When asked about their feelings toward their children or about their qualities as parents, the children of divorce in this study kept talking about being over-protective. They also talked about "caring," "love," "open-mindedness," and "communication"—qualities one would hope all parents have. However, they also mentioned "over-protective," as exhibiting a strong desire to shelter their children rather than make them independent. It was as if they were compensating for a missed childhood.

Discipline is another area that drew some rather consistent responses. Few children of divorce repeated negative discipline habits from their youth. Most aimed to be fair, non-abusive, and consistent. Childhood background meant little in terms of who did the disciplining in a family. The duty of discipline fell to the one who was most present, the one who was more authoritarian, or the one who had a sense of discipline himself.

As Carla explains:

> My current husband is the disciplinarian, even though he's not the kids' father. He has higher standards of discipline and doesn't like my inconsistency. I am sporadic and inconsistent. Even though I deplored that in my mother, I find myself doing the same things.

What adjustments did these children of divorce make as parents because of their parents' divorce? Again, some patterns of conscious behavior appear. One wrote: "I wanted a strong sense of family, togetherness, sharing, and doing. Wanted a strong personal involvement." Another said: "I spent more time doing typical father-son things." And another: "I have a heightened awareness of what a father can do for a son." These comments would not surprise Professor C. John Sommerville, the author of *The Rise and Fall of Childhood*. In correspondence with me, he suggested that this might be the case. He wrote: "I would love to know whether the children of divorce might make more caring and patient parents just because of their experience."

One woman wrote that she gave up her job to watch her children, another recurring theme. Other women, daughters of working mothers, were aware of going home to an empty house after school. They reported making sure they were home when the children were. Some had designed jobs around their children's schedules. This is consistent with research that has found children of divorce with a working custodial parent sometimes perceive the working as a rejection rather than a necessary economic task. Children of divorce try to avoid giving their own children the wrong impression.

Others denied making any conscious adjustments, but added they had a strong sense of family and wanted to ensure continuing family stability. Some parents reported a conscious effort to be models of love, affection, and partnership for their children. Often this conscious effort was exhibited in demonstrative and outward displays of affection between spouses and with children. The family hug is a good example. Even in divorced families, mothers and fathers with their marital relationships broken talked about maintaining good parental relations for the positive development of the children.

Bohannan cites a conversation with a judge about one reason for hostile divorces.

> Donald King, one of the most respected judges in San Francisco, told me that the adversary system works well for litigation such as automobile accidents or contracts, because the contestants need never see one another again, but in child custody cases, the adversary system makes it even more difficult for the parents to communicate afterward.[5]

Kulka and Weingarten support those parents who seek to reduce the trauma of divorce, courts notwithstanding.

> If, in one's childhood experience, divorce comes to be construed as a successful strategy rather than as a personal failure, a potent barrier to leaving a similar stressful situation in one's own adult life could thereby be removed and a more flexible set of coping mechanisms and appreciation for the complexity of relationships could be learned.[6]

Many children of divorce wrote about never establishing relationships with their fathers. Consider Rosemary:

> A few months before he died, my father, from whom my aunt, his only sister, had been estranged for decades, wrote to her. His wife had died, he wondered where I was and whether my children knew about him. She urged me to get in touch with him but I did not. I remembered my grandmother's warning that when he was old, he would look for me to take care of him. (When I had to identify his body on a slab at Bellevue [a New York City hospital], I had not seen him for over 30 years.)

Even reconciliation efforts for children of divorce as adults was difficult or out of the question. In some cases, the mother, implicitly or explicitly, forbade it. In others, the children would not reconcile even if their father desired it. Would you, after 30 years, want to meet the man who "rejected" you as a child? With few exceptions, those who attempted to reconcile with their father found him to be less than the man they expected. He was interested in the children only for what they could do for him after a lifetime of having done nothing for them. Why did some children even bother to attempt reconciliation? Because, as children, they fantasized about their father and what life with him would be like if he were married to their mother and heading their household. When the moment came, they had to find out.

Schlesinger found two themes of reconciliation: either the absent parent would come home or "when the child grew up, he would go and look for the lost parent."[7] Wallerstein and Kelly say: "The poignant fantasies of reconciliation that preoccupied youngsters at every age can be understood as ways of restoring the family in order to help stave off the acute pain of loss."[8]

As adults, children of divorce are always looking back. Wallerstein and Kelly found children of divorce "making continuing comparisons of the present with the past."[9] Additionally, Kulka and Weingarten suggest that coming from a divorced home "may provide a framing experience against which other experiences are consciously or unconsciously measured and, consequently, either pursued or avoided."[10]

Frequently, a child of divorce will compare the present and the past, often to good effect, often so mistakes are not repeated, often to find a baseline of positive behavior. How was something done in the past? With the past as a benchmark of failure, the child of divorce can try a different approach. In effect, the child of divorce has experience.

Others feel the loss of examples. Carol says that her parents' divorce had the biggest effect on her marriage.

I have no examples to fall back on. Nothing to compare, i.e., how would my parents have solved such and such? What would my mother have done in special circumstances? What did my parents do when . . . ? Sometimes I think it must have been easier for my mother to raise her children on her own in her own way rather than with a husband who held a different point of view. Often my husband and I disagree as to what we expect of the children or want of them. Then I think how much easier it was for my mother. Also, I like to make most of the decisions regarding the family simply because my mother did. It surprised me when I first got married that my husband also wanted a part in this. It took a while for me to get used to the idea. This is when I realized how much I really missed with my parents being divorced.

Some children attempt to adopt other families. "As I grew up and went to the homes of friends," Keri recalls,

I used to envy them the presence of a father. In later years I came to realize that though I may have envied the presence of a jolly father or a birthday party, I didn't know about what went on when the party was over. A school friend of over 50 years and I have often discussed this, though her father is one I remember most fondly as she speaks of him with great love.

Laurel remembers one of her friends' family taking her under their wing and trying to help her get over her inferiority feelings.

I even pictured myself belonging to parents of my friends and fantasizing about what life would be like. I stopped doing that after a short time, though, because I accepted the fact that my life was very different from what I would have liked it to be.

To the question of whether children of divorce themselves would consider divorce, the expected answer of "never" does not come as frequently as one would expect. Children of divorce, perhaps because of their experience, would divorce rather than raise their children in a tumultuous environment. Before divorce, however, many would seek counseling. Some stressed a willingness to work a little harder on their marriages and to sacrifice to keep their mate happy. While both men and women were willing to sacrifice, it was primarily the woman, who recognizing her economic vulnerability in a male world, was most willing to take that extra step.

Denise, who is 30 and has been married for 10 years, reflects that attitude.

It always scares me when my husband and I fight. I always think: "Is this it? Is this the biggy that can't be worked out?" In fact, I am so frightened of my husband and I reaching the same outcome that I often find myself apologizing before I really am sorry or even if I wasn't the one in the wrong.

Economic bondage plays a role in keeping woman in unhappy marriages. Lois, 57, remembers her father beating her mother and making Lois and her four brothers and two sisters sleep outside. She did not understand why her mother endured so much before finally leaving. "Mother stated later that she didn't have any money or a place to live and that's why she always tried to live with him. When she couldn't take his beatings anymore, she divorced him."

Other women reported that they would endure a bad marriage as long as there was no violence. "I could never bring myself to leave," says Alice, 41 and a mother of six.

I have been counseled many times. One counselor even found me a place to live, six kids and all, and an emergency welfare check. And I couldn't leave. I figured a part-time father and a nasty grandma (his mom) were better than just one insecure mother. If he wanted to leave, I would never hold him back. I don't know what the future holds but, thus far, I could never leave. I guess I've been there as a kid and it didn't feel good.

Edith, now 56, watched her husband leave once.

When I was married seven years, had two children, pregnant with the third, my husband left me. There were many reasons why he did, but mainly economics (no job), a spoiled child-wife. Not all my fault, but enough. I was frantic. I decided that my children would not grow up without their father and proceeded to work it out. Three months later, after the birth of my son, many concessions on my part and his, we got it together. In retrospect, I thought I had a happy childhood, but when faced with that prospect for my children, it wasn't so great.

By the way, Edith and her husband have now been married for 37 years and have five children.

Still others would stay in an average marriage until the children left the nest. In qualifying their "yes" responses, some parents referred to the trauma divorce can have on children and urged potential divorcers to think of the children first. In defending their "yes" answers, others talked about what a trauma a bad marriage can be for children.

In some instances, the failed marriage of childhood becomes the less than total commitment to the marriage of adulthood. Although married for 17 years and the mother of three children, Romayne still holds back.

> I feel that my parents' divorce made it hard, if not impossible, for me to give total love to a spouse. I can give my children unconditional love because they will always be my children. But who knows if, five or 10 years down the road, I will still be married to the same man. So I cannot give totally to marriage. I am the loser for this. I envy those married people who seem to have total commitment to each other. But I know I can never do it. My father has been married three times. My mother, four times. I am the product from the mother's first and father's second marriage.

Romayne did not mention that a sister who is two years her junior has been married three times.

The ripple effect of divorce can be staggering. Hazel, who is 44 and has been married for 25 years, provided some information on her family:

- I married first; am still married to the same man.
- My mother married twice.
- My oldest sister was married and separated, now deceased.
- My older brother was married four times.
- My younger sister married twice.
- My youngest sister married twice.
- My stepbrother married twice. (He's my stepfather's son from his first wife.)

• My half brother married twice. (He's my brother from my mother and stepfather.)

As Blood puts it, "All human relationships require maturity, but marriage requires more than most."[11]

Although unsolicited, comments on stepparents kept appearing, but they were not consistent. For every child who felt he had been made whole again by a parent's remarriage, there was one who resisted the remarriage and hated the new parent. In some limited circumstances, the child was abused by the new parent. A couple of adults reported not being traumatized by their biological parents' divorce. Instead, they were traumatized by the divorce of their mother and stepfather, for example. In other words, they were affected by the couple that represented the most enduring relationship to the child.

Children of divorce usually miss relationships with a set of grandparents (the parents of the mate who has left) and other relatives. Fran explains it this way:

If asked — "What do I resent most about my situation?" — I would say that I am sorry that other family members did not persist and intervene in my behalf when I was a child. I truly feel I can no longer establish a relationship with my father, and I could not even by the time I was in high school. It disturbs me that aunts, uncles, grandparents on the other side, did not insist that I be known to them. My mother believed she was doing the right thing, but now, as an adult, I think she was very unfair.

Many of the respondents rue the fact that their children will not have a strong relationship with their divorced grandparents. The situation is made worse when both sets of grandparents are divorced. Children of divorce see the value of extended family relationships and mourn their absence. Think of Margaret's earlier comments about the loss of a normal family life for her grandchildren.[12]

No one should be surprised by the differing views siblings have of the same event. You would not expect a 2-year-old to see the same marital discord that a 10-year-old might. You might expect, however, that everyone would have the same perception of the family's economic condition. After all, poor is poor, but again and again among the respondents, siblings remember all aspects of the past differently. I would suggest only that the truth lies somewhere in between. Perception is a fact of life.

As I thought about the subject of divorce before I began my research, I wondered how a child of divorce matures in relation to his peers. I expected that most people would admit what I sense about myself: while growing up I was very mature but, after I grew up, I realized I was not very mature at all. I guess I always mistook independence for maturity. Actually, maturity (in my case) subsequently thrived in a secure environment, not an independent one. Today I feel about 10 years behind my contemporaries. As Peggy puts it:

> Divorced homes had more independent kids who did mature things more often than some others, but I don't think they attained true maturity any sooner. I've always felt I had to be mature and didn't question my true feelings for a long time — well after my marriage. My freedom to grow was curtailed by having to understand even when I didn't and fear of doing wrong and making things worse.

To my surprise, about half the people who answered the questionnaire felt they had matured more quickly than their peers. Look at the comments from the young woman at the beginning of this chapter: "I think I am more independent and more mature as a result."

This is a fairly common refrain. "When I look back on it," says Ray, who is now 43 and in his second marriage, "I probably got a lot of good values like independence, competitive spirit and self-confidence that I might not have gotten otherwise." Wanda, 53, adds:

> I feel I more or less skipped the usual lifestyle of childhood and, from an early age on, was forced by circumstances to act and behave more like an adult than a younger person. Actually, I sometimes feel that maybe part of what I learned from those experiences may have been more beneficial than harm-

ful. I learned early in the game to become a keen observer of much of the real way married people act instead of the way we were taught.

Roseann, whose parents divorced when she was seven, says:

> At the time I didn't realize any difference but later in my teens I found it harder to relate to other kids my own age. Most of the girls my age couldn't cook, knew nothing of running a house or saving and budgeting money, just up in the morning and gone. My mother worked as a core maker in a foundry, so I had chores/jobs to do during the summer months (early in the morning) and I had my afternoons and evenings free. I figured I owed my mom that much and I did it gladly. Boys my age were giddy and frivolous and didn't interest me.

I was also surprised to find only a few children of divorce who had negative experiences with adults other than relatives. I came across research (cited in Chapter One) that showed some divorced women believed janitors scolded their children more sharply because their children had no father at home. I knew the feeling. Yet most respondents reported good or indifferent relationships with adults. Even aunts and uncles (for the most part) were viewed as supportive. The research shows surrogates can serve as alternative sources of affection for father-absent boys.

Scholars who study divorce see it occurring in stages. Linda Bird Francke, like me, is an interested party rather than a primary researcher. She limited her book *Growing Up Divorced* to the first three years after the breakup, although she acknowledged sensing the effects beyond that period. *Parents Whose Parents Were Divorced* has covered the range from one year before the breakup to adulthood. Some may argue that divorce has no impact that far into the future. I disagree. One of the first things that overwhelmed me as I began reading the responses to my questionnaire was the depth of feeling people in their fifties, sixties, and seventies still had about their parents' divorce.

One 45-year-old woman said:

As I matured and became a parent myself, I got very angry about it all. I wanted it behind me but I saw it all in a different light as a parent and I got mad. I was used, I was mistreated, and I was demeaned. I had to live with rotten people in a rotten situation — divorce or no divorce, I was hurt by it.

Said another woman, 44 and married three times ("I'm sorry to say"),

I did not decide to become a parent. I had never wanted to be a parent because of the unhappiness I had experienced all my life. I became a parent because I had no mind of my own, no sense of self-esteem, and when someone told me they loved me and wanted to make love to me, I let them. Why the hell not? I don't think that I ever loved the father of my children. I was incapable of loving anyone as I had no love for myself.

Sometimes the emotion shifts. Anne is 53 and was married for 25 years before she was divorced. She said:

After being shy for many years, the pendulum has swung the other way and I have become very outspoken and can be very nasty at times. I really have to watch myself that I don't get carried away in what I say, especially to my mother. For many years I just let her walk on me, and now I find myself answering her back. Later, I feel badly and upset to think that I have done the things I do, but I never apologize for my actions. I felt like I was suppressed so many years that now it is my turn to speak up.

The childhood experience of divorce hangs over the child of divorce forever, although some struggle to put it behind them. In fact, this may be the single most important thing I have learned: the impact of divorce is everlasting. That does not mean children of divorce go through life flawed, but it does mean that a piece of them is still trying to resolve the trauma of their parents' divorce. Each has his own way of seeking resolution.

As Jill, now 46, explains:

I do recognize that my father had a few good points as a person. It took two psychiatrists and a psychologist to help me work out my anger. I think a dream I had about five years ago can illustrate to you where I now am in my feelings. My father was in a hospital dying. I went to see him. He was very old and sick. He said: "I want you to kiss me." I said: "No, I won't kiss you, but I will hold your hand." And I sat by his side and held his hand as I would for any stranger. I do resent that I never had a real father. It's a void in my life that can never be filled.

Eighteen years after her parents divorced, another woman wrote: "You think that after all these years, you're over the pain and sorrow, but when you start thinking about it all over again it's like an instant flashback. I guess you never really get over it no matter how old you are."

As Samantha's sister Connie puts it: "I still feel guilty about my parents' being divorced. I still try to hide the fact from friends for as long as possible." Connie is now 29.

And then there is denial. In January 1989, an article by Judith S. Wallerstein based on her divorce research appeared in *The New York Times Magazine*.[13] About a month later, the *Times* published a letter from me. That afternoon, my phone rang. I recognized the voice at the other end as that of an elderly woman. She said she was calling to tell me that I was wrong about the impact of divorce. "My parents divorced when I was seven and it didn't have any effect on me. I can remember the day it happened." She went on to describe in some detail the moment her parents decided to divorce. After telling me how wrong I was, she indicated she was not interested in hearing my rebuttal so I never had the chance to point out to her the irony of her phone call.

* * *

Two other matters need to be briefly discussed. How might we minimize divorce and how might we minimize the impact of divorce? For both of these questions, I offer tentative suggestions.

To minimize divorce, Meg and Frances suggest education. "I think in our schools," Meg writes, "they should teach classes in

family life and help people to work for long-term relationships.''
Frances says:

> Divorce is devastating to children and society. There should be
> more education so that people are more prepared for that most
> important step — marriage and children. I have tried to do this
> with my own children.[14]

While to some this may sound like teaching values, I would suggest
that stable marriages undergird a stable society. Or, as Bohannan
puts it,

> We should get our premises straight. The most important one
> for the future is that good families are the ones that make good
> children. The second that good parenthood, not merely a
> happy marriage, is the essence of a good family and of good
> society, no matter what form those families take.[15]

Schools are already responding by recognizing the stress children
of divorce feel and providing counseling. Even college students
now find counseling centers that include experts on divorce. We
help children of divorce through our educational system. Can we
not also use the same system to help children avoid divorce when
they become adults?

When divorce is necessary, how can we minimize its impact?
More and more schools are developing courses in divorce and providing counseling services for children of divorce. We seem to be
taking the right steps in reducing the emotional impact of divorce on
children. However, such efforts cannot work alone. We cannot reduce the emotional stress unless we also reduce the economic
stress. As one respondent put it, ''Support laws should be worked
on; we had a terrible time financially.''

Here is one woman's analysis of the effect of her mother's divorce:

> My mother is 71 years old, on Social Security, has very little
> money. We help support her, which is not really fair to my
> husband because we could make other investments (he doesn't
> complain, though). I still resent my dad for that today because

her care has fallen on the kids and I'm the only one financially able to help. She appreciates all we do and is very independent and would starve before she would ask for anything, but common sense shows she can't live on Social Security. She still works part-time in a school cafeteria. I feel that being married 20 years and [having] five kids, the court should have made him have an insurance policy or something to provide for her care being she never remarried.

Some researchers have suggested that the negative impact of a father's absence could be diminished if wives without husbands in the home had some economic stability.[16] The problem becomes more acute with age. Schlesinger says that women who divorced after 30 usually remain divorced while divorced men are more likely to remarry.

Because of the assumption that divorcees will remarry, society does not feel obligated to provide supports for single parents. Because societal supports are largely unavailable, husbandless mothers come to view remarriage as the only viable alternative to a difficult situation. The situation will remain difficult as long as policies are based on these circular assumptions.[17]

Two other researchers speak of an institutional bias against one-parent families that perceives them to be either as flexible as two-parent families or as abnormal.[18] The system established to protect people ends up exploiting them. It is as though social Darwinism rather than humanism dominates our society. We force some people to live on the fringe of society and then we establish support systems to help them. However, these same support systems keep these people on the fringes rather than helping them back into the mainstream.

And why not? It is more profitable. In Bohannan's words, "A well-family industry isn't as profitable as a divorce industry. So services to one-parent families or stepfamilies run from scarce to nonexistent."[19] Lawyers alone receive a total of $3 billion a year for handling divorce cases. Add to that the costs for ancillary services: marriage and divorce mediators, special attorneys, property appraisers, accountants, private investigators, and therapists. In 1980, about 700 lawyers concentrated on divorce. In 1985, the number was 11,000.[20] As long as society is unwilling to help one-parent homes, the negative effects of divorce will probably linger for a long time.

At the very least, we need to get a grip on the economic problem. Mitigating the negative impact of the sudden drop in income may help. Schorr offers a solution to the economic problem:

> Children deprived of a parent because of divorce or legal separation would receive benefits under the general conditions and scale of payments that apply to survivors' insurance. Application would be made by the parent who cares for them.[21]

Terry Arendell also argues for job training, flexible work schedules, child care programs, health insurance and pension coverage, and housing and centralized community resources.[22] This does not mean that the economically stronger spouse would not contribute. Since Schorr is suggesting a federal program, it seems simple to add that the economically stronger spouse could make mandated payments through his Social Security deduction. That might get at the problem of spouses who skip town and never pay support.[23]

We need to help the people who are most vulnerable in a divorce. We must recognize who suffers and for how long. With the number of divorces rising, we must address its impact squarely. Divorce is more than an individual problem; it is a problem for our society.

ENDNOTES

1. Hetherington, Cox, and Cox in Lamb, *Nontraditional Families: Parenting and Child Development*, p. 252.
2. Laiken, p. 72.
3. Glenn, p. 69.
4. Kulka and Weingarten, p. 56.
5. Bohannan, p. 25. (Undoubtedly adding to the contentious nature of the proceedings was the court's attempt to fashion a reasonable joint custody agreement. California, which once considered joint custody the preferred approach, has changed its mind, according to an article in the December 1988 issue of *Governing* magazine.)
6. Kulka and Weingarten, p. 76.
7. Schlesinger, *Journal of Divorce*, p. 11.

8. Wallerstein and Kelly, pp. 46-47.

9. Ibid., p. 197.

10. Kulka and Weingarten, p. 58.

11. Blood, p. 162.

12. An element I had not examined arose after I completed this manuscript: grandparents who act as parents while their divorced child works. My mother called this phenomenon to my attention by sending me an article about a former friend of mine who, with her husband, was parenting one of their granddaughters.

13. The article, "Children After Divorce," was adapted from *Second Chances: Men, Women and Children a Decade After Divorce* by Judith S. Wallerstein and Sandra Blakeslee, published in 1989 by Ticknor & Fields.

14. My files contain news stories about a variety of high school courses on marriage. Unfortunately, some have to be geared to the needs of students whose parents are divorced, but other schools are able to offer courses as preparation for marriage. I took a course in college titled "Courtship and Marriage," but I'm afraid that, because it was a large lecture course, its potential was never reached. For such a course to have an impact, students need to role play and act out situations under the guidance of professors.

15. Bohannan, p. 235.

16. Hetherington, Cox, and Cox in Lamb, *Nontraditional Families*, p. 245.

17. Schlesinger, *Journal of Divorce*, p. 4.

18. Thompson Jr., Edward H., and Gongla, Patricia A., "Single-Parent Families: In the Mainstream of American Society" in Macklin and Rubin, p. 114.

19. Bohannan. p. 16.

20. Weglarz article in *The Wall Street Journal*. Sources cited in the article include Paul Bohannan, the American Divorce Association for Men and Women, the American Divorce Association, and the American Bar Association.

21. Schorr, p. 115.

22. Arendell, p. 160.

23. As this book was going to press, a federal law guaranteeing financial support for children of divorce was being phased in. Legislators learned it was cheaper to ensure that fathers made court-mandated support payments than to run a welfare system.

Bibliography

Academic Articles

Ahrons, Constance R., and Bowman, Madonna E., "Changes in Family Relationships Following Divorce of Adult Child: Grandmother's Perceptions," *Journal of Divorce*, Vol. 5, Nos. 1/2.

Biller, Henry B., and Bahm, Robert M., "Father Absence, Perceived Maternal Behavior and Masculinity of Self-Concept Among Junior High School Boys," *Developmental Psychology*, Vol. 12, No. 4, 1976.

Bonkowski, Sara E.; Boomhower, Sara J., and Bequette, Shelly Q., "What You Don't Know Can Hurt You: Unexpressed Fears and Feelings of Children from Divorcing Families," *Journal of Divorce*, Vol. 9, No. 1, Fall 1985.

Burchinal, Lee G., "Characteristics of Adolescents from Unbroken, Broken, and Reconstituted Families," *Journal of Marriage and the Family*, Vol. 26, No. 1, February 1964.

Cain, Barbara S.; "Parental Divorce During College Years" in *Psychiatry*, Vol. 52, No. 2., 1989.

Fine, Mark A.; Moreland, John R., and Schwebel, Andrew I., "Long-Term Effects of Divorce on Parent-Child Relationships," *Developmental Psychology*, Vol. 19, No. 5, 1983.

Hagestad, Gunhild O.; Smyer, Michael A., and Stierman, Karen L., "Parent-Child Relations in Adulthood: The Impact of Divorce in Middle Age," chapter prepared for *Parenthood: Psychodynamic Perspectives*, 1982.

Henderson, Keith, "A Prep Course on Marriage," *Etc.*, Vol. 44, No. 1, Spring 1987.

Herzog, Elizabeth, and Sudia, Cecelia E., "Fatherless Homes: A Review of Research," *Children*, September-October 1968.

Hodges, William F., and Bloom, Bernard C., "Parent's Report of Children's Adjustment to Marital Separation: A Longitudinal Study," *Journal of Divorce*, Vol. 8, No. 1, Fall 1984.

Jellinek, Michael S., and Slovik, Lois S., "Divorce: Impact on Children," *The New England Journal of Medicine*, September 3, 1981.

Kaslow, Florence, and Hyatt, Ralph, "Divorce: A Potential Growth Experience for the Extended Family," *Journal of Divorce*, Vol. 5, Nos. 1/2.

Keith, Pat M., and Schafer, Robert B., "Correlates of Depression Among Single Parents, Employed Women," *Journal of Divorce*, Vol. 5, No. 3, Spring 1982.

Kemper, Theodore, "Predicting the Divorce Rate," *Journal of Family Issues*, Vol. 4, No. 3, September 1983.

Kinard, E. Milling, and Reinherz, Helen, "Marital Disruption," *Journal of Family Issues*, Vol. 5, No. 1, March 1984.

Kitson, Gay C., and Raschke, Helen J., "Divorce Research: What We Know; What We Need to Know," *Journal of Divorce*, Vol. 4, No. 3, Spring 1981.

Kulka, Richard A., and Weingarten, Helen, "The Long-Term Effects of Parental Divorce in Childhood on Adult Adjustment," *Journal of Social Issues*, Vol. 35, No. 4, 1979.

MacKinnon, Carol E.; Stoneman, Zolina, and Brody, Gene H., "The Impact of Maternal Employment and Family Form on Children's Sex-Role Stereotypes and Mother's Traditional Attitudes," *Journal of Divorce*, Vol. 18, No. 1, Fall 1984.

Martin, Teresa Castro and Bumpass, Larry L., "Recent Trends in Marital Disruption," *Demography*, Vol. 26, No. 1, February 1989.

McDermott, John F. Jr., "Parental Divorce in Early Childhood," *American Journal of Psychiatry*, Vol. 124, No. 10, April 1968.

Morgan, S. Philip; Lyne, Diane N., and Condran, Gretchen A., "Sons, Daughters, and the Risk of Marital Disruption," *American Journal of Sociology*, Vol. 94, No. 1, July 1988.

Nye, F. Ivan, "Child Adjustment in Broken and in Unhappy Unbroken Homes," *Marriage and Family Living*, November 1957.

Pett, Marjorie G., "Correlates of Children's Social Adjustment Following Divorce," *Journal of Divorce*, Vol. 5, No. 4, Summer 1982.

Pett, Marjorie G., "Predictors of Satisfactory Social Adjustment of Divorced Single Parents," *Journal of Divorce*, Vol. 5, No. 3, Spring 1982.

Russell, Ivan L., "Behavior Problems of Children from Broken and Intact Homes," *The Journal of Education Sociology*, Vol. 31, No. 3, 1957.

Santrock, John W., and Warshak, Richard A., "Father Custody and Social Development in Boys and Girls," *Journal of Social Issues*, Vol. 35, No. 4, 1979.

Schlesinger, Benjamin, "Children's Viewpoints of Living in a One-Parent Family," *Journal of Divorce*, Vol. 5, No. 4, Summer 1982.

Sexton, Thomas L.; Hingst, Ann G., and Regan, Kathleen, "The Effect of Divorce on the Relationships Between Parental Bonding and Sexrole Identification of Adult Males," *Journal of Divorce*, Vol. 9, No. 1, Fall 1985.

Smyer, Michael A., and Hofland, Brian, "Divorce and Family Support in Later Life," *Journal of Family Issues*, Vol. 3., No. 1, March 1982.

Sorosky, Arthur, "The Psychological Effects of Divorce on Adolescents," *Adolescence*, Spring 1977.

Spanier, Graham B., and Glick, Paul C., "Marital Instability in the United States: Some Correlates and Recent Changes," *Family Relations*, July 1981.

Spanier, Graham B., and Hanson, Sandra, "The Role of Extended Kin in the Adjustment to Marital Separation," *Journal of Divorce*, Vol. 5, Nos. 1/2, Fall/Winter 1981.

Thomes, Mary Margaret, "Children with Absent Fathers," *Journal of Marriage and the Family*, February 1968.

Thornton, Arland, and Freedman, Deborah, "Changing Attitudes Toward Marriage and Single Life," *Family Planning Perspectives*, Vol. 14, No. 6, November/December 1982.

White, Lynn K.; Brinkerhoff, David B., and Booth, Alan, "The Effect of Marital Disruption on Child's Attachment to Parents," *Journal of Family Issues*, Vol. 6, No. 1, March 1985.

Popular Articles

Bohannan, Paul, "The Binuclear Family," *Science 81*, November 1981.

Brandt, Anthony, "Father Love," *Esquire*, November 1982.

Bridgewater, Carol Austin, "Divorce: The Long-term Effects on Children," *Psychology Today*, July 1984.

Cain, Barbara S., "Older Children and Divorce" *The New York Times Magazine*, February 18, 1990.

Collins, Glenn, "Redefining the Role of Fathers," *The New York Times*, June 14, 1983.

Dullea, Georgia, "How Women Fare in No-Fault Divorce," *The New York Times*, November 7, 1985.

Dullea, Georgia, "If Parents Part: Young Adults Describe Their Own Anguish," *The New York Times*, November 11, 1985.

Duscha, Julius, "The Kids They Leave Behind," *The Washington Post*, June 20, 1982.

Francke, Linda Bird, "Children of Divorce," *Family Circle*, July 12, 1983.

Francke, Linda Bird, "The Surprising Joys of Single Parenthood," *The Washington Post*, November 1, 1981.

Fuchs, Victor R., "Divorce Rate's Fiscal Impact," *The New York Times*, September 7, 1983.

Glenn, Norval D., "Children of Divorce," *Psychology Today*, June 1985.

Goleman, Daniel, "Patterns of Love Charted in Studies," *The New York Times*, September 10, 1985.

Goleman, Daniel, "Clues to Behavior Sought in History of Families," *The New York Times*, January 21, 1986.

Hellmich, Nanci, "Kids of Divorce Don't Count on Reunions," *USA Today*, February 3, 1986.

McDermott, John F., Jr., "Divorce from Three to Six," *The New York Times Magazine*, October 22, 1977.

Mincer, Jilian, "L. I. Counselor Helps Children Deal with Shock of Divorce," *The New York Times*, July 1, 1985.

Schmid, Randolph E., "Study: Divorce to Teach Record for Women in Their 30s," Associated Press story in the *Centre Daily Times*, State College, Pennsylvania, April 5, 1986.

Sherman, Beth, "Helping the Child of Divorce," *The New York Times*, April 14, 1985, Section 12, p. 20.

Wallerstein, Judith S., and Blakeslee, Sandra, "Children After Divorce," *The New York Times Magazine*, January 22, 1989.

Weglarz, Nilda R., "Divorce Becomes a Big Business As Cases Grow in Size, Complexity," *The Wall Street Journal*, August 28, 1985.

Whitmer, Margaret, "When a Marriage Falls Apart," Port Huron, Michigan, *Times Herald*, January 26, 1984.

Books

Arendell, Terry, *Mothers and Divorce: Legal, Economic, and Social Dilemmas*. Berkeley: University of California Press. 1986.

Berelson, Bernard, and Steiner, Gary A., *Human Behavior: An Inventory of Scientific Findings*. New York/Burlingham: Harcourt, Brace & World, Inc. 1964.

Blood, Robert O., Jr., *Marriage*. Second Edition. New York: The Free Press. 1969.

Bohannan, Paul, *All the Happy Families: Exploring the Varieties of Family Life*. New York: McGraw-Hill Book Company. 1985.

Cherlin, Andrew J., *Marriage, Divorce, Remarriage*. Cambridge, Massachusetts, and London, England: Harvard University Press. 1981.

Cull, John G., and Hardy, Richard E., eds., *Deciding on Divorce: Per-*

sonal and Family Considerations. Springfield, Illinois: Charles C Thomas. 1974.

Francke, Linda Bird, *Growing Up Divorced*. New York: Fawcett Crest. 1983.

Greif, Geoffrey L., *Single Fathers*. Lexington, Massachusetts: Lexington Books, D.C. Heath Company. 1985.

Harding, Esther, M., *The Parental Image: Its Injury and Reconstruction*. New York: G.P. Putnam's Sons. 1965.

Hoffman, Lois Wladis; Gandelman, Ronald, and Schiffman, H. Richard, eds., *Parenting: Its Causes and Consequences*. Hillsdale, New Jersey: Lawrence Erlbaum Associates. 1982.

Laiken, Deidre S., *Daughters of Divorce. The Effects of Parental Divorce on Women's Lives*. New York: William Morrow and Company, Inc. 1981.

Lamb, Michael E., ed., *The Role of the Father in Child Development*. New York: John Wiley & Sons. 1981.

Lamb, Michael E., ed., *Nontraditional Families: Parenting and Child Development*. Hillsdale, New Jersey: Lawrence Erlbaum Associates. 1982.

LaRossa, Ralph, and LaRossa, Maureen Mulligan, *Transition to Parenthood: How Infants Change Families*. Beverly Hills and London: Sage Publications. 1981.

Laswell, Marcia E., and Laswell, Thomas E., eds., *Love, Marriage, Family*. Glenview, Illinois: Scott, Foresman and Company. 1973.

Lauer, Robert, *Social Problems and the Quality of Life*. Dubuque, Iowa: William C. Brown Co. 1982.

Leslie, Gerald, *The Family in Social Context*. New York: Oxford University. 1979.

Levinger, George, and Moles, Oliver C., eds., *Divorce and Separation: Context, Causes and Consequences*. New York: Basic Books, Inc. 1979.

Luepnitz, Deborah Anna, *Child Custody: A Study of Families After Divorce*. Lexington, Massachusetts: Lexington Books, D.C. Heath and Company. 1982.

Macklin, Eleanor D., and Rubin, Roger H., eds., *Contemporary Families and Alternative Lifestyles*. Beverly Hills and London: Sage Publications. 1983.

Masnick, George, and Bane, Mary Jo, *The Nation's Families: 1960-1990*. Boston, Massachusetts: Auburn House Publishing Company. 1980.

Norwood, Robin, *Women Who Love Too Much*. Los Angeles: Jeremy P. Tarcher, Inc. 1985.

Olson, David H.; McCubbin, Hamilton I.; Barnes, Howard; Larsen, Andrea; Muxen, Maria, and Wilson, Marc, *Families: What Makes Them Work*. Beverly Hills and London: Sage Publications. 1983.

Roberts, Albert R., ed., *Childhood Deprivation*. Springfield, Illinois: Charles C Thomas. 1974.

Schlesinger, Benjamin, *The One-Parent Family: Perspectives and Annotated Bibliography*. Toronto: University of Toronto. 1978.

Schorr, Alvin L., *Poor Kids: A Report on Children in Poverty*. New York/London: Basic Books, Inc. 1966.

Sears, Robert R.; Rau, Lucy, and Alpert, Richard, *Identification and Child Rearing*. Stanford, California: Stanford University Press. 1965.

Sommerville, C. John, *The Rise and Fall of Childhood*. Beverly Hills and London: Sage Publications. 1982.

Stuart, Irving R., and Abt, Lawrence Edwin, eds., *Children of Separation and Divorce*. New York: Gossman Publishers. 1972.

Stuart, Irving R., and Abt, Lawrence Edwin, eds., *Children of Separation and Divorce: Management and Treatment*. New York: Van Nostrand Reinhold Company. 1981.

Thamm, Robert, *Beyond Marriage and the Nuclear Family*. Canfield Press: San Francisco. 1975.

Udry, J. Richard, *The Social Context of Marriage*. Philadelphia: J.B. Lippincott Company. 1966.

Wallerstein, Judith S., and Kelly, Joan Berlin, *Surviving the Breakup: How Children and Parents Cope with Divorce*. New York: Basic Books Inc. 1980.

Weiss, Robert S., *Going It Alone: The Family Life and Social Situation of the Single Parent*. New York: Basic Books Inc. 1979.

Weiss, Robert S., *Marital Separation*. New York: Basic Books Inc. 1975.

Weitzman, Lenore J., *The Divorce Revolution*. New York: The Free Press. 1985.

Wilkerson, The Reverend David R., with Cox, Claire, *Parents on Trial: Why Kids Go Wrong—Or Right*. New York: Hawthorn Books. 1977.

Monographs

Ianni, Francis A.J., *Home, School and Community in Adolescent Education*. New York: ERIC Clearinghouse on Urban Education. Institute for Urban and Minority Education, Teachers College, Columbia University.

Kirchner, Elizabeth P., and Seaver, W. Burleigh, with the assistance of

Margaret K. Straw and Maria E. Vegega, *Development Measures of Parenthood Motivation*. University Park, Pennsylvania: Institute for Research on Human Resources.

Reports

Gingsburg, Alan, "Single Parents, Working Mothers, Socioeconomic Status, and Children's Achievements," (working draft), U.S. Department of Education. June 1983.

Marital Status and Living Arrangements: March 1981. U.S. Department of Commerce, Bureau of Census. Washington, DC: U.S. Government Printing Office. 1982.

Marital Status and Living Arrangements: March 1983. U.S. Department of Commerce, Bureau of Census. Washington, DC: U.S. Government Printing Office. 1983.

Marital Status and Living Arrangements: March 1986. U.S. Department of Commerce, Bureau of Census. Washington, DC: U.S. Government Printing Office. 1987.

Marital Status and Living Arrangements: March 1987. U.S. Department of Commerce, Bureau of Census. Washington, DC: U.S. Government Printing Office. 1988.

Marital Status and Living Arrangements: March 1988. U.S. Department of Commerce, Bureau of Census. Washington, DC: U.S. Government Printing Office. 1989.

The State of Families 1984-85. New York: Family Service America. 1984.

Appendix

A QUESTIONNAIRE FOR CHILDREN
OF DIVORCE WHO ARE NOW PARENTS

To the respondent: The purpose of this questionnaire is to obtain opinions and attitudes. There are no right or wrong answers.

This questionnaire is broken into five parts that try to reflect different aspects of your life. Isolating each aspect is, of course, impossible so you may encounter a question in the "wrong" category. Please answer it anyway. Every effort has been made to organize this questionnaire in a logical way to make answering it as easy as possible. In some cases, it was necessary to list responses to questions in columns in order to save space.

The five parts of this questionnaire are: I. Personal Information. II. Former Family Information. III. Childhood Information. IV. Custodial and Non-custodial Parent Information. V. Current Parental Information.

I. Personal Information

1. Today's Date _____

2. Name _____   Sex: Male   Female
   Address_____
           (number and street)

   _____
       (town, state, and zip code)

3. Telephone ( ) _____

4. Date of Birth _____ / _____ / _____
           day   month   year

5. Circle your ethnic group:

   A. White
   B. Black

   C. Spanish American
   D. Native American
   E. Other (specify) _____

6. Circle your marital status:

   A. married*
   B. separated

   C. divorced
   D. widowed

   * If it is your second marriage, please check here ___

7. How many years have you been married: ____

8. How old were you when you and your spouse married:

   A. you _____   B. spouse _____

9. What are the ages of each of your children:

   _____   _____   _____   _____   _____   _____

10. Circle your religious preference:

    A. Roman Catholic
    B. Protestant

    C. Jewish
    D. Agnostic / Atheist
    E. Other (specify) _____

11. Circle the response that best describes your personal
    church attendance:

    A. weekly
    B. almost weekly

    C. monthly
    D. holidays
    E. never

12. Circle the highest level of education you attained:

    A. some high school
    B. high school / technical

    C. some college
    D. bachelor's degree
    E. graduate / professional degree

13. Evaluate your educational achievements through high school (if appropriate) by circling one response:

A. superior   C. average
B. above average   D. below average
                     E. inferior

14. Frequently we hear someone say that a person is more like one parent than the other. Usually, the person is referring to looks, personality, temperament, or habits. Which parent are you now more like and why do you feel this way?

15. What is your present occupation? _____

[End of Part I]

II. Former Family Information

To the respondent: Many of the questions you will be asked in this section deal with your parents' divorce. Because I am interested in when their marriage effectively ended (that is, when they stopped living together), I would call that the time of the divorce rather than the time a judge signed the divorce decree. For example, my parents separated when I was five years old but did not divorce until I was in my early 20s. For my purposes here, my parents divorced when I was five years old.

1. How old were you when your parents divorced? _____

2. How many brothers did you have? _____

3. How many sisters did you have? _____

4. How many of your sisters / brothers were older? _____

5. How many of your sisters / brothers were younger? _____

6. Describe your family life one year before your parents divorced.

7. How long were your parents married at the time
    of their divorce? _____

8. A. How did you find out about your parents' divorce?

    B. Describe your reaction.

9. Why did your parents divorce?

10. Check the response that best describes your parents' church attendance before they divorced:

	Father	Mother
A. weekly	___	___
B. almost weekly	___	___
C. monthly	___	___
D. holidays	___	___
E. never	___	___
F. don't recall	___	___
G. don't know	___	___

11. Describe your relationship with each parent before they divorced.

Father

Mother

12. Try to recall how you felt about each parent before they divorced. What qualities did they have?

Father

Mother

13. A. If after your parents divorced, you and your custodial parent lived with your grandparents, please answer Part B of this question. If not applicable, check here and continue to question 14. _____

  B. During the first years you lived with them, describe your relationship with your grandparents.

  <u>Grandfather</u>

  <u>Grandmother</u>

14. A. Check the highest level of education that your parents had attained by the time of their divorce.

	Father	Mother
A. some high school	_____	_____
B. high school / technical school	_____	_____
C. some college	_____	_____
D. bachelor's degree	_____	_____
E. graduate or professional degree	_____	_____

  B. If that changed at any time after the divorce, what did it change to?

	Father	Mother
A. some high school	_____	_____
B. high school / technical school	_____	_____
C. some college	_____	_____
D. bachelor's degree	_____	_____
E. graduate or professional degree	_____	_____

15. What were your parents' occupations at the time of their divorce?

    A. Father _____

    B. Mother _____

16. What were your parents' approximate ages when they married each other?

    A. Father _____   B. Mother _____

[End of Part II]

III. Childhood Information

<u>To the respondent:</u> The questions in this section expect you to give an opinion or attitude that you held *after* your parents effectively divorced, not before.

1. Describe your relationship with your brothers and/or sisters.

2. Describe your relationship with your childhood friends after your parents divorced.

3. Describe the effect your parents' divorce had on how you matured compared to how your friends matured.

4. Describe how adults other than relatives treated you after your parents divorced.

5. Describe how your aunts and uncles treated you after your parents divorced.

6. Describe your attitude toward unrelated adults after your parents divorced.

7. Describe your attitude toward your aunts and uncles after your parents divorced.

8. Describe the image you had of yourself growing up in a divorced home.

[End of Part III]

IV. Custodial and Non-custodial Parent Information

To the respondent: Two terms used in this section may need to be clarified. The *custodial parent* is the one who provided a home for you and your brothers and sisters and lived with you after your parents divorced. The *non-custodial parent* was not present in the home.

1. After your parents divorced, which parent retained custody?

   A. Father   B. Mother   C. Other (specify) _____

2. What was your family's economic standard of living under your custodial parent?

3. Circle one response in each column below to describe the type of community you and your custodial parent lived in after your parents divorced:

Population

A. up to 15,000
B. 15,001 - 40,000
C. 40,001 - 100,000
D. 100,001 - 500,000
E. more than 500, 000

Description

F. large city
G. small city
H. suburb
I. small town
J. rural

4. What was your custodial parent's work status within one year after the divorce?

5. What was your non-custodial parent's work status within one year after the divorce?

6. How would you characterize the way your custodial parent disciplined you?

7. What kind of person was your custodial parent?

8. How frequently did your non-custodial parent visit you in the first year after your parents divorced?

9. If that frequency changed, when did it change and to what did it change?

10. What did you and your non-custodial parent do when your non-custodial parent visited?

11. How did your non-custodial parent behave toward you during these visits?

12. How did you feel toward your non-custodial parent?

13. How would you characterize the way your non-custodial parent disciplined you?

14. Describe your parent's relationship one year after they divorced.

[End of Part IV]

V. Current Parent Information

1. How do you feel toward your children?

2. What qualities do you see in yourself as a parent?

3. What adjustments have you made in raising your children because you grew up as a child of divorce?

4. In your family, who is the major source of discipline for your children and why?

5. How would you characterize the way you discipline your children?

6. A. Compare yourself as a child and your oldest child in the following categories and check which describes your oldest child. (After each word, put a check mark or X in the appropriate column; you should have only one answer per word):

	Better	Worse	Same
behavior	____	____	____
possessions	____	____	____
luck	____	____	____
friendships	____	____	____
relation with grandparents	____	____	____
education	____	____	____
family	____	____	____
parents	____	____	____

B. If you want to comment on any of your responses to 6. A., please do so here:

7. Evaluate your oldest child's educational achievements through high school (if applicable) by circling one response.

   A. superior   C. average
   B. above average   D. below average
                          E. inferior

8. What kind of a relationship do your children have with their <u>divorced</u> grandparents?

9. How did you explain your parents' divorce to your children? How old were they?

10. How do you feel your parents' divorce affects your children?

11. When you decided to become a parent, did your parents' divorce affect your decision? If it did, how?

12. If you felt your marriage was no longer working, would you divorce your spouse or grant your spouse a divorce? Why or why not?

13. Please use the following space to comment on any area not covered in this questionnaire.

14. If you think any of your brothers and/or sisters would participate in this project, please provide their names and addresses so they can be sent the questionnaire. Please remember that all responses will be kept confidential.

[End of Part V]

END OF QUESTIONNAIRE

Thank you very much — R. Thomas Berner

Index